DEATH BY
PRESCRIPTION

DEATH BY
PRESCRIPTION

THE SHOCKING TRUTH BEHIND AN OVERMEDICATED NATION

Ray D. Strand, M.D.

with Donna K. Wallace

OLIVER
NELSON

THOMAS NELSON PUBLISHERS
Nashville

A Division of Thomas Nelson, Inc.
www.ThomasNelson.com

Published in Nashville, Tennessee, by Thomas Nelson, Inc.

Scripture quotations are from the NEW AMERICAN STANDARD BIBLE®, © Copyright The Lockman Foundation 1960, 1962, 1963, 1968, 1971, 1972, 1973, 1975, 1977. Used by permission.

Published in association with the literary agency of Alive Communications, 7680 Goddard Street, Suite 200, Colorado Springs, CO 80920.

Library of Congress Cataloging-in-Publication Data

Strand, Ray D.
  Death by prescription : the shocking truth behind an overmedicated
nation / Ray D. Strand, with Donna K. Wallace.
      p. cm.
Includes bibliographical references and index.
  ISBN 0-7852-6484-1 (hardcover)
  1. Drugs—Side effects—Prevention—Popular works. 2. Medication errors—Popular
works. 3. Drugs—Toxicology—Popular works. 4. Drug approval—United States—
Popular works. I. Wallace, Donna K. II. Title.

RM302.5.S775 2003
615'.7042—dc21   2003013641

Printed in the United States of America
02 03 04 05 06 BVG 5 4 3 2 1

CONTENTS

This book is dedicated to the most precious of my gifts—
my children: Donny, Nick, and Sarah. You have brought me great joy.

Introduction

I YAWNED WITH FATIGUE AND FELT MY EARS POP AS I ADJUSTED to the cabin pressure in the airplane. Loosening the seat belt, I leaned back, attempting to rest my head in spite of the jarring vibration of the twin engines. Harried events of the past forty-eight hours played out in my mind like disjointed reruns. I hadn't noticed the sterile smell of antiseptic in the air ambulance on my previous ride, but now as the plane returned to my hometown, I kept swallowing and shifting restlessly. The air felt tight.

A little blonde girl with big round eyes now lay in a children's hospital connected to tubes and IVs, fighting for her life. She had almost died during transport. I glanced at my watch, wondering if Heidi was still alive. Hers was not an anonymous face; Heidi was *my* patient—the child of a close friend.

Wiping the sweat from my brow, I prayed yet again for healing and for mercy. You see, Heidi was not the victim of a drunk driver or a serious illness. An adverse drug reaction to a medication I had prescribed for her was threatening her life.

Nothing in medical school or my postgraduate education had prepared me for this. Feelings of helplessness and frustration washed over me, and I kept seeing her eyes pleading, "Doctor, please help me." Was the tremor in my stomach from the vibration of the plane, or a deep shaking of my confidence? I wanted to quit, run away, never again have to face another sick child or parents desperate for answers. I was exhausted.

I may have dozed off. I'm not sure if I was asleep or awake, but undoubtedly, I sensed a voice whisper deep within saying, "Come to Me, all who are weary and heavy-laden, and I will give you rest" (Matt. 11:28). "Cast your cares upon Me." As I repeated these words over and over, they began to fill me, and I was able to relax and breathe freely. This personal message of God's compassion for all who are afflicted has since carried me through many years of medical practice and now through the pages of this book.

I don't anticipate a book such as this being a big hit in the medical community. But since that evening flight high above the South Dakota plains, my heart has grown fiercely protective of young and old alike. I will do whatever it takes to relieve pain and suffering for people of all ages.

Heidi couldn't read the plaques in my office that spelled out my awards, licenses, and medical degrees. She was not aware of the volumes of scientific research I had pored over late at night. She might never comprehend the politics involved in the lengthy and complicated processes of drug approval and the FDA's role in protecting her from the very event that threatened to crush her. This little child certainly couldn't recognize the hundreds of medical staff members needed for her care. Heidi simply wanted to live.

Medical training, much like that of military personnel or policemen and firemen, teaches us to distance ourselves from emotional crises that can arise in our work. We must remain strong, no matter what degree of trauma we see. Statistics and technical jargon help to dull potential distress in the medical community, but the opposite reality also rings true.

Medical statistics represent faces. I have based this book on research statistics, but I have written about real people. Every statistic on these pages represents a life: a mom, a dad, grandma, a close friend, son, or daughter. When I cite cases of those injured from adverse reactions to drugs, I recall the faces and families of my patients who've come into my office with similar concerns. When I learn of a young woman who lost her life just by taking the combination drug Fen-Phen, I can imagine the despair in her husband's eyes. These are real-life scenarios.

As I reflect back over my thirty years of family practice, I have studied and witnessed both the pitfalls and successes of medicine and what they mean for families everywhere. Today, modern medications seem to have taken their place on "hallowed ground." If I had titled this book *Death by Heart Attack* or *Death by Cancer*, I doubt anyone would balk. After all, teaching patients how to prevent a heart attack or avoid developing cancer is acceptable and good medicine. But teaching patients how they can avoid the number-three killer, adverse-drug events, steps on some toes. Whether politically correct or not, I will go where few choose to tread. Someone must address the life and death issue of *death by prescription*. Don't you agree?

Thus, this book. You will find in Part I the fascinating history and inner workings of the drug approval "system" as it stands today. In Part II, I explain how and why the system has gone wrong and illustrate with real-life scenarios of drugs that have been pulled from the market. You may be surprised to learn the rest of the story about dangerous drugs you recognize or may even have taken. Part III provides an insider's view from the physician's stance on practical guidelines so that you can assess *how great* your risk is and make appropriate decisions about your medication needs.

In this book I focus again on the task set before me: not only to help relieve pain, but to empower you in protecting and regaining your health. Together may we prevent yet another *death by prescription*.

PART I

THE "SYSTEM"

CHAPTER ONE

Death by Prescription

WITH A SHIVER CYNTHIA PUT ON THE LITTLE GOWN THAT gaped open down the back. Not too anxious to climb up on the paper-lined exam table, she opted instead to perch on the edge of a short stool while she waited for her doctor to come in. It wasn't cold in the little room, but the patient wrapped her arms tightly around her middle. Over the years Cynthia had become accustomed to her annual gyne-cological checkup and pap smear, but it would be a stretch to say one ever became comfortable with them.

She had learned years ago that the best way to pass the time in these little rooms was to close her eyes, breathe deeply, and recall her many bless-ings one by one. She had so much for which to be thankful. At age forty-eight, Cynthia was truly living the life for which most women yearn.

Deep breath in, slow exhale out. Deep breath in . . . scenes of mother-hood, a lovely home, dear friends, and a partnership shared with her husband in real estate and development flipped through her mind like pages in a family photo album. Some of her favorite blessings were the kids, of course. "Lord, thank You!" she whispered.

The youngest of their three children had just gone away to college, and now she and Phil were looking forward to a new chapter with

3

more freedom—one filled with travel and adventure. Raising three teenagers had given her a few strands of gray hair, but Cynthia remained in excellent health as a result of eating right and staying fit.

Over the last six months, Cynthia had started having night sweats and hot flashes, so she wanted to discuss menopause with her doctor during this visit. She would explain to him that her periods had been getting farther apart and that she had actually missed one entirely a couple of months ago.

After listening carefully and doing a thorough exam, the doctor confirmed that Cynthia was indeed entering menopause and strongly encouraged her to start hormonal replacement with estrogen and progestin. With confidence he explained the tremendous benefits of taking hormone replacement therapy (HRT), with the assurance that estrogen would improve all of her menopausal symptoms. He also claimed that HRT would decrease Cynthia's risk of developing osteoporosis, Alzheimer's dementia, heart attack, and stroke. HRT could even improve her sex life.

Of course, Cynthia was in favor of actively defending her body against such diseases, but she'd always believed that being a good steward of her health was sufficient. Noticeably hesitant, Cynthia questioned the doctor about possible risks of taking hormone replacement therapy. She was not excited about taking *any* type of medication—especially for the rest of her life.

The soft-spoken physician leaned forward and insisted that every woman needed hormonal replacement and that it was *essential* for her to take it over the long term. Glancing over Cynthia's chart, the doctor said that HRT could increase her risk of developing breast cancer. But the medical literature had some conflicting reports as to whether or not this was true, and he felt the findings were inconclusive.

With a tone that brought the discussion to a close, the doctor said, "The benefits of taking hormonal replacement far outweigh any risks you may encounter. In the hundreds of patients I've treated, never once have I seen any complications related to HRT."

Cynthia was obviously intimidated, and in the end she consented to accept his recommendations. After all, she was paying for professional advice and wanted to do everything possible to protect her health. Faithfully she began taking her estrogen and progestin each day. She was relieved when her hot flashes and night sweats began to diminish and finally disappeared completely. Soon she also added some calcium and vitamin D supplements to her daily regimen and continued her work-out program. Months passed, and she was feeling great.

———

Cynthia woke up to sunshine and birds singing. The thermometer read 72 degrees, and she had spring-cleaning in mind. For starters, she would open the doors and windows for some fresh air, then she'd do some thorough scrubbing and cut a bouquet of tulips and daffodils for the foyer.

Suddenly Cynthia felt an unusual, crushing heaviness in her chest. She became short of breath and began sweating profusely. The chest discomfort first spread to her left shoulder and then down her left arm. Phil was not home, so she half-crawled, half-dragged herself over to the phone and dialed 911. Cynthia was beginning to lose consciousness and couldn't form any words. Within seconds, she crumpled to the floor.

With the phone line still connected, the 911 operator was able to trace the call and alert the paramedics. Within fifteen minutes they arrived and found Cynthia lying on the floor. The paramedics started cardiopulmonary resuscitation and rapidly transported her to the nearby hospital emergency room.

The ER physician and entire emergency room staff set to work immediately in a frantic attempt to save Cynthia's life. The reception staff located Phil and informed him about what was happening. Dropping everything, he raced to the emergency room. But when he arrived he was not allowed to go back to the room where his wife lay, still totally unresponsive. Straining, he could see at least a half-dozen people working to resuscitate his wife. He recognized his friend Paul, a local cardiologist, who had been making his morning rounds and had responded to the "code blue" announced over the hospital's intercom system. Phil was gripped in shock and disbelief.

Another twenty-five minutes of gut-wrenching waiting passed after a nurse had ushered Phil to a private family waiting room close to the ER. Just when he thought he could not wait a minute longer, he looked up, and there stood his friend Paul. By the drawn look on Paul's face, Phil knew the report was not good.

Paul spoke with a quiver in his voice, "Phil, Cynthia is dead—we tried everything to save her, but we just could not get a response."

Phil sat in total disbelief. He tried to make sense of the words he'd just heard, but he could see only his wife's face that he'd kissed before leaving for work just two hours before. She had been vibrant and full of energy.

"Phil, she suffered a heart attack and went into cardiac arrest—her heart just stopped. We tried everything to get it beating again, but nothing helped."

The Rest of the Story

Weeks passed after the tragic morning that forever changed Phil and his family's life. Cynthia was gone, and the loss filled every waking moment of their lives. They had consented to an autopsy and learned that indeed, she had died of an acute coronary thrombosis—a heart attack. The news was baffling, because Cynthia didn't have any risk factors for heart disease. In fact, she was physically active, watched her diet closely, and even had normal cholesterol levels. There was not even a recorded history of heart disease in her family. Phil finally decided to go to lunch with his cardiologist friend Paul to get some answers.

His friend wasn't very talkative at lunch, but after some casual, courteous remarks, Phil asked the cardiologist for his opinion. "Why? Why did Cynthia suffer a heart attack?"

After a long pause, Paul carefully informed Phil that he believed Cynthia's heart attack was most likely due to the hormone replacement therapy that she had started several months earlier. Paul went on to say, "Estrogen is known to cause an increased risk of developing blood clots and subsequent embolism to the legs, lungs, or brain." Recent clinical studies had actually shown an increased risk for heart attacks and strokes in women on hormonal replacement, especially during the first year, he added.

Phil was confused. "I distinctly remember Cynthia saying that one of the reasons the gynecologist put her on the hormones in the first place was to decrease the risk of heart attack and stroke!"

The cardiologist shook his head as he responded, "This is what we have thought for years. But in the past year or so studies have revealed this increased risk of heart attacks is probably greater than any of us could have before imagined or anticipated." He concluded, "I am truly sorry."

> Cynthia's heart attack was most likely due to the hormone replacement therapy that she had started several months earlier.

More questions bombarded Phil's mind. *This is a risk of estrogen that has been known for the past year or so . . . known for the past year? By whom? The maker of the drug? The doctor who prescribed it? The pharmacist who filled the prescription?* Why were he and Cynthia the last to know? If recent clinical studies had shown an increased risk for heart attacks and strokes in women on hormonal replacement, what was it doing in Cynthia's medicine cabinet? And why had the gynecologist actually told Cynthia that one of the reasons he wanted her to take it was to decrease her risk of heart attack and stroke?

Injuries and deaths like Cynthia's are not simply statistics. Each one marks a family that suffers a tremendous and unexpected loss. If only Phil and Cynthia had realized the potential danger of hormonal replacement therapy. After all, menopause is not a disease; it is simply a stage of life. Phil now realizes that this adverse drug reaction does not occur often; however, he also knows that when it happens to *you*, percentages don't really mean much. As far as he is concerned, this adverse drug reaction may as well happen 100 percent of the time.

A Report That Rocked the Medical Profession

You may be tempted to think that Cynthia's story is rare happenstance, and the chance of you or someone you love having a similar experience is almost nonexistent. Even as a physician I would have agreed with you until 1998, when I encountered a shocking article in the prestigious *Journal of the American Medical Association (JAMA)*. The article was titled "Incidence of Adverse Drug Reactions in Hospitalized Patients."

There the authors reviewed thirty-nine studies detailing adverse drug reactions documented in U.S. hospitals over the past thirty years. They determined, even by very conservative analysis, that in 1994 more than 2.2 million people required hospitalization because of serious reactions to medications. Even more troubling was the fact that more than 106,000 of these patients actually died because of adverse drug reactions—reactions to properly prescribed and administered medications. The authors of the *JAMA* article concluded that these totals have not changed significantly over the past thirty years.[1]

This report exploded like a bomb in the medical profession. We had no idea the number of patients affected by adverse drug reactions was so high. Physicians were so filled with disbelief that many of them questioned the integrity of the report and its data. The authors, however— all doctors themselves—had gone to great lengths to make sure their conclusions about adverse drug reactions were credible. Their data stood the test. Because they had excluded all questionable cases, their estimated numbers were low, not high.

Why are these numbers so shocking? Other than the personal heartache connected with the death of each of these people, is this really a big deal? It *is* a big deal. Let me put the numbers into context: the number-one killer in the United States is heart disease—around 743,000 deaths each year. The number-two killer is cancer, which accounts for 529,000 deaths. Number three is strokes, which total about 150,000 deaths annually. Guess what the number-four killer is? Is it automobile accidents or AIDS? No, each of them claim only 41,000 lives every year.[2] America's number-four killer is adverse drug reactions to *properly* prescribed medication, with more than 100,000 estimated deaths per year. And if you add the 80,000 deaths caused by *improperly* prescribed or administered medication, adverse drug events become the *number-three* leading cause of death in this country.[3] In comparison, 56,000 people were killed during the ten years of the Vietnam War and just under 3,000 people were killed on September 11, 2001, by terrorist attacks. Now you can understand why the *JAMA* article caused such a tide of unbelief!

Doctors and patients alike see drugs as a huge contributor to health. We wonder, then, *how can it be that this favored tool in medicine is actually a significant foe for thousands of innocent patients?* To say the least, this is a terribly disconcerting finding, because we doctors love our drugs. I'll explain why.

The Making of a Doctor

The anticipation I felt as I entered my first year of medical school in 1967 was overwhelming. I was one of the few students who had been accepted into medical school following my junior year of college. I had worked hard, and now it was all paying off. This was the beginning of my dream; becoming a medical doctor would give me the lifelong opportunity to truly help people. Any challenges to come would be well worth the effort.

My second year of medical school was especially memorable because I was finally able to take classes that I felt would really prepare me to be a doctor. After taking rudimentary courses of biochemistry and physiology my first year, now I would study pathology and pharmacology. Physicians being disease-oriented and pharmaceutically trained, I remember my excitement as I learned about all the different medications. Doctors need to know a lot about drugs—namely, how the body absorbs and excretes them. With great enthusiasm I learned when and how I should use each drug. Of course, we eager medical students had to learn the specific side effects and dangers of each as well.

Drugs are synthetic, which means they are not natural to the body. Every drug inevitably affects a natural enzyme system within the body to accomplish a therapeutic result. Most of the time the body completes this process successfully—no big deal. Problems with drugs arise, however, because each drug *also* affects other enzyme systems in ways that may be harmful. The inherent problem with medications is that no one can know all the possible problems drugs may cause.

In my medical training I concluded that the harmful side effects of drugs were rare, and usually mild, occurrences. One bit of advice did stick in the forefront of my mind, though. My professor of pharmacology emphasized over and over, in regard to prescribing medication, "First, do no harm!" What he meant was, "Always consider whether the potential risk of a drug outweighs any potential benefit for the patient."

I am certain every medical student receives a similar warning. But like most doctors, I was so intent on helping patients and using medication to accomplish that goal, I didn't think too much about the potential danger of drugs. When patients came to me with their complaints, I would think primarily of the possible diseases they might have contracted. I rarely, if ever, considered the possibility of a drug reaction causing their problems. On occasion, especially in cases of patients on antibiotics, I would encounter an allergic reaction to a medication. Yet these instances were typically not serious.

Several years into my medical practice, however, one patient's case changed forever the way I thought about prescription drugs. This man, a prominent businessman in my community, had high blood pressure. To treat his hypertension I prescribed medication from an exceptional class of new drugs called *angiotensin converting enzyme inhibitors*—now called ACE inhibitors.

Sometime later he came to see me because of a dry, hacking cough that had persisted for several weeks. At times the man coughed so hard it literally took his breath away. These coughing spasms were so brutal and painful that he had to leave the room and bring the coughing under control in private. I examined him and ordered a chest x-ray. To my surprise, the x-ray was normal, and he didn't have any evidence of pneumonia or any other lung problem.

Stumped by his symptoms, I referred the man to a pulmonary specialist who did a complete battery of tests but could not determine a diagnosis either. Three other lung specialists in the same clinic then saw this patient and were not able to conclude what was wrong. We tried various antibiotics and asthma medications. Nothing helped.

After he had suffered six months of almost continual coughing, I referred him to the pulmonary department at the University of Minnesota. Again he went through another round of extensive tests. Still no definitive diagnosis explained the coughing.

When I saw my patient in my office a few months later, he was beyond miserable. He could hardly speak a sentence before breaking into harsh, persistent hacking. He had decided to retire and move south for the winter, hoping to find relief.

About five months later I received a short note from a resident physician who had evaluated this man at the University of Minnesota. Attached to the letter was a clipping from a medical journal. The article reviewed a case in which a patient with an unexplained cough was taking an ACE inhibitor medication for high blood pressure. When the patient in the article quit taking the drug, the cough disappeared.

The resident who sent me the article had remembered my patient and his horrible cough, as well as the fact that he was taking an ACE inhibitor high blood pressure medication. The physician suggested that we try switching the patient's medication, and see what happened to the cough.

I called my patient immediately and advised him to switch to a high blood pressure prescription from a different class of drugs. In the eighteen months of taking the ACE inhibitor, this man had not had an hour without a coughing spell, but to our amazement his cough quit within a week or two after he discontinued its use. The culprit was the high blood pressure medication.

All those pulmonologists and I had no clue that a side effect of these drugs could cause such a cough. When the drug was tested in clinical trials prior to approval for public use, a bad cough had not surfaced as a side effect. Now physicians realize that a cough is a common side effect of ACE inhibitor blood pressure medication.

How many patients like mine suffered so much, for so long?

Adverse Drug Events

An entirely different category of drug reactions exists, and they are called adverse drug *events*. An adverse drug event is an injury resulting from *medical intervention* related to a drug. This not only includes injuries that occur from properly prescribed medications but also those injuries to patients resulting from errors in the way their physicians prescribed or administered medications. Such errors include prescribing the wrong drug or the wrong dosage, and giving a medication by mistake to the wrong person. This category also includes injuries caused when patients have taken their medications improperly.

The really tragic part of this scenario is that several studies indicate that nearly half of these adverse drug events are preventable.[4] As I mentioned earlier, in a 1995 *JAMA* article, Dr. David Bates estimated that adverse drug events cause approximately 180,000 deaths each year.[5] Kent Nelson, a doctor of pharmacology, stated, "Almost one-half of these adverse drug reactions were definitely avoidable . . . If inappropriate prescribing was responsible, efforts to educate physicians could have a major impact. However, physician errors accounted for only 5% of the adverse drug-related admissions. The high rate of [patient error] suggests that a patient-centered strategy for decreasing the problem may be more effective."[6]

Several studies estimate that 5 percent of all hospital admissions are the result of an adverse drug event.[7] And the odds of a problem with medication increase once a person enters the hospital—where the average patient receives ten different drugs during a hospital stay. Those most critically ill, some studies have shown, receive upwards of thirty-eight different drugs during their hospitalizations![8] The greater the number of drugs a patient requires, the greater the risk of experiencing an adverse drug event. Simply stated, the more drugs you use, the greater the chance of error—and the greater the chance of an adverse drug event.

The FDA—Our Protector?

You may be thinking, *That is all very interesting, but don't we have the government working to protect us from this kind of thing? Aren't prescription drugs rigorously controlled?*

The answer to those questions is "Yes—*but* . . ." The U.S. government's Food and Drug Administration (FDA) is doing its best to protect you from danger related to drugs, but the job is really an impossible one. The FDA operates at a busy and dangerous intersection where a number of often-competitive interests collide. What was once considered to be one of our greatest protectors has now formed a deadly partnership with the pharmaceutical industry. If you are presently taking medication or plan to use any drugs in the future, you need to become more knowledgeable about the use and inherent danger of drugs. After all, it may save your life or the life of a loved one. Having blind faith in the FDA, your doctor, or your pharmacist may prove to be costly. As you read this book, you will begin to realize that you are a key player in a chain of events in preventing a serious adverse drug reaction. Therefore, a basic understanding and awareness of the players involved in this chain of events is a necessity to avoid the third leading cause of death in this country.

> You need to become more knowledgeable about the use and inherent danger of drugs. After all, it may save your life.

When a drug provides the desired result, everyone is happy. But when the drug has an unwanted result, a tragedy can and will occur. Who is responsible for the drug's final outcome? The entire chain of players. A medication's ability to bring about proper results is dependent on

- the pharmaceutical company's clinical studies during the drug's approval process;
- the FDA's regulatory actions and nonactions;
- the doctor's decision to prescribe the medication;
- the pharmacist's filling of that script;
- and last but not least, the patient's ability to take the medication as directed.

Though this chain of events has been in place for nearly fifty years, weighty decisions have been subtly shifted to the final link in the chain. Health-care professionals are placing the decision-making about patients' health into the hands of patients themselves. Placing blind trust in the Food and Drug Administration is no longer a sufficient choice.

Potent drugs are also now available over the counter, placing heavy responsibility of self-care on each individual. Although we realize the dangers of illegal drugs, we must now learn the pitfalls of living in a broader drug culture. Ours is a society in which the expanding number of medications continues to multiply exponentially with each passing year.

What is the solution to this largely unreported aspect of America's health crisis?

Take Charge of Your Health

Certainly, improvements can and should be made in the system of approving new drugs and monitoring adverse drug reactions. We all need to support efforts in the public and private sectors to bring about positive change; still, the most important person in protecting your health from a harmful or even fatal encounter with a prescription drug is *you*. This is something you can and should do now. Don't expect the FDA, your doctor, or anyone else to take full responsibility for your greatest natural resource—your health.

Why am I so adamant that you must become the chief guardian of your health? First, the medical care system in America has changed radically. We now depend on outpatient treatment far more than in the past. Between 1983 and 1993 the number of outpatient visits in the United States increased by 75 percent, while during the same time the number of hospital inpatient days fell by 21 percent.[9] Because of the skyrocketing cost of care, physicians now only admit patients to the hospital who either need major surgery or who are suffering from a serious illness or injury. Furthermore, they send hospitalized patients home as quickly as possible.

> The most important person in protecting your health from a harmful or even fatal encounter with a prescription drug is *you*.

Second, as a result of this medical care environment, we physicians are using more potent drugs than we did even a few years ago. Studies also reveal how doctors are having more difficulty in maintaining continuity of their patients' care with the growing trend of specialized care. Both these trends have contributed to increased medication errors and, in turn, increased adverse drug events. Patients are seeing so many different physicians that their medical care is becoming fragmented, and too many times there is really no particular physician in charge.[10]

The bottom line is that patients must know their drugs and be much more actively involved in their treatment, fully understanding that every time they take a medication there is a risk. Medical experts who research this growing epidemic are confident, as I have said, that we can avoid more than half of the injuries and deaths due to adverse drug events. But who is educating the most important player in this chain of events—you? This book is really at the center of preventive medicine; and anyone who is currently taking medication or plans to in the future needs to read it.

> It is absolutely imperative that you know the dynamics that play against each other to make prescription drugs a major threat to your health.

Over the years I've developed a deep respect for the medications I prescribe. While in active, private family practice for over thirty years, I've seen the use of properly prescribed medication help thousands of patients. And I continue to prescribe medications to my patients on a daily basis. But I have also gained great insight into the dangers of all drugs and believe physicians should use them as a *last resort rather than a first choice*.

Again, every time a physician writes a prescription, he or she must essentially weigh the inherent risk of the drug against the possible benefits for the patient. Though health-care professionals can prevent many of the deaths and injuries medications cause, this is not a simple, cut-and-dried process. You, too, must weigh your risks against your benefits with a thorough understanding of how the FDA approves drugs and how adverse drug reactions are reported. It is absolutely imperative that you know the dynamics that play against each other to make prescription drugs a major threat to your health.

CHAPTER TWO

The Drug-Approval Process

MIKE AND I HAD MANY THINGS IN COMMON. LIKE ME, HE LOVED golf and the great outdoors, and he was a devoted family man. Even with a bustling home with four little children, he and Julie were involved at their church. They were especially gifted at helping other couples with troubled marriages.

I admired Mike for his aggressive approach to business while holding fast to integrity and honor. At age thirty, he stayed in excellent shape not only physically, but spiritually and relationally too. He seemed to live the balanced life for which we all strive.

In the middle of September, the young dad came down with a head cold that just about knocked him out. He figured he could fight it off and spent the next ten days taking over-the-counter antihistamines and cold remedies. In spite of good rest and lots of fluids, Mike only got worse. When he developed a fever of 102 degrees coupled with severe pressure in his sinuses, Julie grew worried and made an appointment for him with their family doctor that afternoon.

The doctor evaluated him and diagnosed an acute sinus infection. He asked Mike if he was allergic to any antibiotics, and Mike answered that he was not. Instead of writing a prescription, his doctor went over to the sample meds cabinet and pulled out a ten-day supply of a new antibiotic a pharmaceutical representative had left just the day before. The doctor explained that this was a new quinolone antibiotic called Raxar. Usually he would prescribe amoxicillin, but Raxar, a new drug that the FDA had approved a little over a year prior, was stronger and the price was right—*free*. He asked Mike to call him back in about three or four days if he wasn't feeling better.

Mike started taking the sample antibiotics, and within a few days he had definitely gotten better. But on the sixth day of antibiotics, he started to feel odd. He came home during his lunch break, thinking he would lie down for a little bit before going back to the office. After resting briefly, he sat up on the couch and called for his wife in the kitchen:

"Julie! Julie, I don't . . . feel right."

At the urgency in his voice, Julie left the children at the table eating their macaroni and cheese, and ran into the living room.

"What is it? What doesn't feel right?"

Shaking, Mike sat on the edge of the couch. He felt light-headed, he told his wife, as if he might pass out. Julie hurried to get a cool washcloth for his face.

Two minutes later, her husband collapsed to the floor and was unconscious. Terrified, Julie called 911 while she pleaded,

"Mike! Mike! Sweetie, answer me! Please! What's wrong?"

He was not responding at all. Julie looked for the emergency procedures she kept by the refrigerator. Two-year-old Hannah was crying, and the other children sat frozen, not knowing what to do.

Although it took only ten minutes for the ambulance to arrive at their home, it seemed to Julie like an eternity. In transport to the emergency room, paramedics began CPR but could not get a response. They administered intracardiac epinephrine under the direction of the ER physician, but still there was no response.

A mere forty-five minutes after the paramedics first arrived, they pronounced Mike dead. His new widow and children huddled together in the emergency room, crying and praying. In an instant, their husband and daddy had been taken away.

Julie decided to have an autopsy performed for the sake of the children's health. Mike's doctor felt that a cardiac arrest must have been the result of a heart attack. If this were true, Julie felt the children could be at risk of developing the same problem in the future, and she needed to know for certain.

Thousands of patients die each year taking medication for minor medical problems.

The autopsy results were a complete surprise. Mike's heart was perfectly normal and showed absolutely no evidence of coronary artery disease. In fact, the coroner's report listed the cause of death as a cardiac arrest *secondary* to Raxar, the antibiotic he had been taking the past week. The coroner could find no other cause of death.

You can imagine my response as Mike's friend when just two months after his death, the FDA removed Raxar from the market. It turned out that the drug had been suspected in several deaths caused by fatal heart-rhythm disruptions. I then followed the Raxar issue closely and found reports stating there was evidence in the preclinical trials of fatal heart-rhythm disruptions. Interestingly, the FDA officials chose to exclude any mention of the deaths from the drug's label when it released Raxar to the public.

My research didn't help Mike, but it can help you. No one considers the fact that an antibiotic prescribed for a simple upper respiratory infection and sinusitis could potentially cost someone his life. We often believe that if a patient dies from a serious adverse drug reaction it is because the patient was already very ill and probably would have died in a few months anyway. The truth is, however, that thousands of patients die each year taking medication for *minor* medical problems.

Safe and Effective

Safe. Effective. What comes to mind when you hear these two words? When I hear the word *safe,* I think of protection—being out of harm's way. I envision children safe in their beds, or jewels locked securely in a safe. Its partner, *effective,* means success. An effective team, for instance, is competent and efficient. Couple these two words together, and bind them to a promise on a drug label or advertisement, and we feel totally at ease. Why shouldn't we?

When the Food and Drug Administration approves a drug for distribution to the general public, it states it has found this drug to be "safe and effective." Without a doubt, this leads the medical community and the public to gain a sense of confidence in the medication. When we open a prescription bottle and pull out the tuft of cotton on top, we believe we are about to swallow the most suitable drug designed for our needs and that it will heal our bodies.

You must know, however, that the FDA's definition of *safe* is not the same as it is for you and me. In fact, nothing could be further from the truth. Because of the inherent nature and risk of drugs, absolutely no drug is ever completely safe.

For those of you who are taking prescription meds, you may be feeling nervous or frightened about this. None of us wants his sense of security threatened. You may even be wondering, *Why do we have the FDA, and what does it do for me?*

> Because of the inherent nature and risk of drugs, absolutely no drug is ever completely safe.

Most Americans are at least vaguely familiar with the organization that serves as our protector . . . but what is it really? How has the FDA evolved? What does it actually do? Let's take a look. The history and processes of the FDA will help us better understand our nation's dilemma with prescription medications.

From the Annals of History

The issue of how best to regulate the safety and effectiveness of pharmaceuticals has always been a concern of Congress. We can trace this mission back to the year 1906, the year Congress passed the first drug law—The Food and Drugs Act. This was great progress, yet this new law required only that drugs meet standards of strength and purity.[1] A pill had only to contain the exact dosage stated on the bottle and the exact drug that appeared on the label. The burden of proof still rode on the shoulders of the government to prove a drug's label as false and/or fraudulent before it could be taken off the market. This was a start, but it obviously did little to protect patients.

Later, a bill was introduced in the Senate to completely revise the 1906 drug law, but congressional action was stalled. It may come as no surprise that it took a tragedy, in which more than one hundred people died from a poisonous ingredient, to promote passage of the revised legislation. Historical documents record that the tragedy came about when a solution called Elixir Sulfanilamide had been mislabeled an "elixir," implying that it was an alcoholic solution. Instead, it was a diethylene-glycol mix, an untested poisonous new drug formulation.[2] Drug safety quickly became a priority for Congress.

Prompted by the deaths the poisonous substance caused, Congress passed the Federal Food and Cosmetic Act (FDCA) in 1938. This action led to the establishment of the FDA as we know it today. The FDCA gave the FDA the authority to develop regulations and to actually *control the flow of drugs into the marketplace*. For the first time in history, the newly established FDA required drug manufacturers to prove that their drugs were safe prior to marketing.[3]

Did you know that it wasn't until Congress passed the Durham-Humphery Amendment in 1951 that a drug could be labeled "For Sale by Prescription Only"? (Many of my patients, and perhaps you, too, remember that year. It was not so long ago.) This amendment determined that a drug would be defined "a prescription drug" when it was determined unsafe for self-medication and meant for use only under the direction of a physician.[4]

As more and more drugs became available, our dependence on the FDA increased. The FDA has since grown into one of the few bureaucracies that the public generally supports. But Americans' faith in its protective regulator didn't take its giant leap forward until after a terrifying international event known as the Thalidomide Tragedy.

Thalidomide: The *Titanic* of the Pharmaceutical Industry

The *Titanic* has become the metaphor for the disastrous consequences of our untainted belief in the safety and invincibility of technology. Made even more famous by the multimillion-dollar movie by the same name, the story of 1,500 people who lost their lives when the "unsinkable" ship went down in the North Atlantic conjures up images of fear and dispels our once-free trust in modern engineering. Believed to be the safest passenger ship of its time, the *Titanic* sank to its doom because of human error and overreliance on technology.

The sunken ship, the *Titanic,* has surely become a symbol of all great disasters in our time. Just as surely, the drug thalidomide is the *Titanic* of the pharmaceutical industry. The Thalidomide Tragedy of the late 1950s and early 1960s forever changed how we view the safety of medicines and their potential dangers. Thalidomide terrified Americans, and we ran to the arms of safety and protection of the FDA. This marked the shift of our trust in science to an unwavering reliance on this agency.

Thalidomide was first introduced to Germany in 1958 as an anticonvulsive drug, but physicians soon found it unsuitable for that particular use. They recognized early on, however, that the drug offered other benefits, such as relief from morning sickness caused by pregnancy. By 1961, they prescribed thalidomide for morning sickness all across the continent of Europe. Pregnant women in forty-eight countries used thalidomide during their pregnancies.[5] Of the infants that were exposed to thalidomide between days 35 and 48 after their mothers' last menstrual period, 20–30 percent were born with severe limb and organ defects.[6]

> It was a tragedy of unequaled proportions, because it was the fault of innocent, unknowing mothers taking a drug for a minor problem during pregnancy.

I vividly remember seeing a baby on the front cover of a major magazine with no legs, and arms that were developed only down to the elbows. An image that will forever be imprinted on my mind, this helpless infant was one of more than eight thousand that thalidomide impacted. It not only affected limbs, but almost every organ in their tiny bodies, including the heart, gastrointestinal tract, liver, and urinary tract. It was a tragedy of unequaled proportions, because it was the fault of innocent, unknowing mothers taking a drug for a minor problem during pregnancy. Had they known the risks involved, no European mother would have ever considered taking thalidomide.

Thalidomide failed to receive FDA approval and was never released in the United States. This fact alone produced tremendous credibility for the FDA. Breathing a huge sigh of relief, we found our faith tightly reinforced in the drug-approval process that the FDA governed. The Food and Drug Administration had certainly proved itself to be our great protector.

The irony of this tragic situation is that the FDA had initially withheld approval of thalidomide in the United States not because of severe malformations in infants, but because it had caused some nerve damage in people who were taking the medication. Simply put, we were lucky. In the United States, only seventeen infants suffered the effects of thalidomide. This number is astonishing after we learn that its manufacturer had distributed 2.5 million tablets to American physicians to be used in clinical trials. The FDA quickly halted use of the drug by American physicians when the news of the horrors of thalidomide became known.[7]

The Thalidomide Tragedy not only ended the popular medical belief that the sanctuary of the uterus protected the human fetus from maternal exposure to drugs, but it also ushered in the greatest change of drug regulation in the history of the United States.

Society was dumbstruck when an iceberg brought ruin to a vessel of safety. The incident forever marred the world's trust in ship technology. And when a drug infiltrated the haven of a mother's womb and caused unprecedented harm, the world's eyes were opened to the potential inherent risk of medication. What first appeared to be a random mishap soon became of widespread international concern. The world looked on with a newfound apprehension for safety.

News reports about the role of the FDA keeping the drug thalidomide off the U.S. market aroused great public interest in drug regulation.[8]

Congress successfully passed the Kefauver–Harris Drug Amendments in 1962. These amendments were intended to tighten up control on drugs.[9]

Now pharmaceutical companies had to prove not only the *safety* of their drugs, but their efficacy for the diseases they were intended to treat. These amendments required pharmaceutical companies to send all reports of possible adverse drug reactions of their medications to the FDA, and the pharmaceutical industry now had to provide complete information to doctors detailing not only the *benefits* of the medication, but also the *risks* of taking the medication. This drug information is what we now refer to as the *drug label* or *drug information package insert*.

New Drug Development Process

When it comes to illnesses, none of us would choose a difficult road to travel. The road has twists and turns with unexpected dangers, and we can never be certain of the stops along the way or the sights we'll see. My ultimate goal is to show you how to get off a road filled with potholes and ruts, and find a smoother road to health. But for now you must become familiar with the vehicle you're in, so that when you are confronted with a decision whether or not to take a drug, you'll know better what to do.

I believe it is *vitally* important for people to understand the basic process for getting a drug approved by the FDA. Taking a prescription is like buying a used car. You want to know where it's been and what it might do before you set out on a long trip. By learning what is involved in the drug development process, you will be able to determine your personal needs and be able to steer away and protect yourself from a serious adverse drug reaction.

Believe it or not, few physicians or people in the general public are fully aware of all that is involved in getting a drug approved. Drug approval in the United States requires a carefully planned series of steps, sometimes taking as long as twelve years to complete, and it involves billions of dollars and numerous industries and professionals such as chemists, research specialists, medical professionals, lawyers, politicians, marketers, and pharmaceutical reps. It was estimated that in 1998 the pharmaceutical industry spent $24 billion dollars in research and development alone.[10]

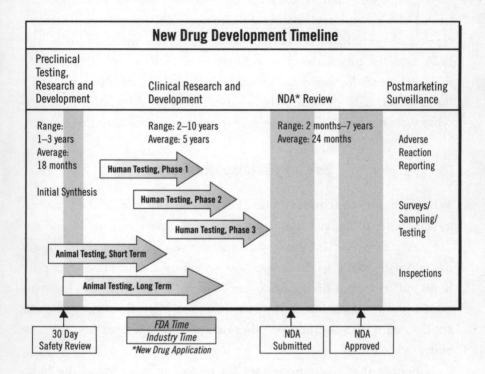

New Drug Development Timeline

Preclinical Testing, Research and Development	Clinical Research and Development	NDA* Review	Postmarketing Surveillance
Range: 1–3 years Average: 18 months	Range: 2–10 years Average: 5 years	Range: 2 months–7 years Average: 24 months	Adverse Reaction Reporting
Initial Synthesis	Human Testing, Phase 1		
	Human Testing, Phase 2		Surveys/ Sampling/ Testing
	Human Testing, Phase 3		
Animal Testing, Short Term			Inspections
Animal Testing, Long Term			

30 Day Safety Review

FDA Time
Industry Time
*New Drug Application

NDA Submitted

NDA Approved

Research and development is a major expenditure for the pharmaceutical industry, with an estimated 20 percent of sales from its drugs going back into research and development.[11] This money is primarily spent for the purpose of getting drugs through the FDA's multiphased approval process. The process first begins with preclinical research done on animals, followed by a new drug application to the FDA. The third step involves three phases of testing on humans. Next, the FDA committee reviews the completed drug application and must make a decision on whether it should approve the drug or not.

Following is a more detailed explanation of each step.

> Taking a prescription is like buying a used car. You want to know where it's been and what it might do before you set out on a long trip.

Preclinical Research

A pharmaceutical company first synthesizes and develops a new drug compound. After finding a compound that has potential, the company then begins to produce larger amounts of the drug. It is initially concerned about its purity and quality. Research scientists will then begin testing the drug in a laboratory—most likely in cell cultures and with animals—to identify the drug's toxic effects and pharmaceutical action.

Animal testing of the drug is the next step. The FDA requires that any drug needing its approval must first be tested in at least two different animal species. It is here that investigators learn how the drug is absorbed and eliminated (for example, through the liver or kidneys) and its potential pharmaceutical and toxic effects.[12]

The purpose of the preclinical trials is to develop adequate information about the drug and so determine the safety of proceeding to human trials with the drug. The FDA usually requires a safety review of the information gathered during the animal trials before allowing the company to begin testing its drugs in humans.

New Drug Application

When a pharmaceutical company has identified a promising drug during the preclinical trials, it will then apply for a New Drug Application (NDA) through the FDA. This NDA must provide reviewers at the FDA with sufficient information to reach several key decisions such as

- whether the drug is safe and effective for its proposed use, and whether the benefits of the drug outweigh its risks.
- whether the drug's proposed labeling is appropriate.
- whether the methods used in manufacturing the drug and the controls used to maintain the drug's quality are adequate to preserve the drug's identity, strength, quality, and purity.

The NDA usually occurs once the company is comfortable with the safety and effectiveness of its drug noted during the animal trials.

Testing on Humans

Clinical trials with humans represent the ultimate premarket testing ground for unapproved drugs. During these trials investigators give a new drug to humans and evaluate it for its safety and effectiveness in treating, preventing, or diagnosing a specific disease or condition. The results from these trials will comprise the single most important aspect in the approval or disapproval of a new drug.[13]

In medicine's most celebrated clinical trial, Louis Pasteur treated patients who had been exposed to rabies with an experimental antirabies vaccine. *All of the treated patients survived.* It was obvious that his treatment was effective, since everyone knew that this disease was 100 percent fatal. This, however, is a very unusual case—drugs do not typically reverse a fatal illness.

Determining a drug's effectiveness is an arduous task, primarily because diseases do not typically follow a predictable path. Many acute illnesses, such as viral infections, minor injuries, and headaches, will usually go away spontaneously (on their own). And most chronic degenerative diseases, such as multiple sclerosis, arthritis, asthma, and lupus, have varying courses. In other words, there are times the patient may do better and times the patient may do worse as a normal progression of his disease. There is no way to predict these changes in the patient's clinical course. These complicated and perplexing dynamics often make it very difficult to be absolutely sure that any drug is effective and actually improves the overall course of a disease.

Controlled Clinical Trials

The FDA relies primarily on controlled clinical trials to determine whether a drug is effective or not. In a controlled trial, patients in one group receive the investigational drug while a control group receives a placebo (a sugar pill made of an inactive substance that looks like the investigational drug). The dynamics of these groups are as similar as possible.

Most clinical trials are designed in such a fashion that the investigators and the patients do not actually know if they are getting the drug or the placebo. This arrangement, called a *double-blind study,* eliminates any possible bias the patient or the investigator may have. It is also common practice to *randomize the patients* (meaning investigators select patients randomly and assign them to either the control group or a treatment group). Such a process of selecting subjects for the study ensures that no patient is deliberately selected for one group or another. (This is an important point to remember if you ever consider getting involved in a clinical trial: You may or may not receive the investigational drug.) Investigators of the clinical trial must remain as objective as possible. These controlled clinical trials are then categorized as Phase 1, Phase 2, or Phase 3 Clinical trials.[14]

Phase 1 Clinical Trials

At this stage, the investigators' main goal is to clarify what happens to a particular drug within the human body. They closely monitor people in a Phase 1 Clinical Trial, and these trials usually involve only healthy subjects. *The number of subjects involved with these studies varies, but is usually small, generally in the range of twenty to eighty people.*

Phase 1 studies determine how well the body absorbs the drug and how it actually gets rid of it, either through the kidneys or liver. In a typical testing period of about three to six months, Phase 1 studies also determine side effects associated with increasing doses of the drug and may even give early evidence of the effectiveness of the drug. These studies usually do not reveal major problems with a drug, such as unacceptable adverse drug reactions or toxic effects on the body.

The FDA observes Phase 1 Clinical Trials closely and works with pharmaceutical companies in the design of future clinical trials. If the agency is concerned about any aspects of the drug at this point, it may put a hold on further testing in humans. If, on the other hand, the new drug still appears promising, the FDA will approve it for further investigation in Phase 2.

Phase 2 Clinical Trials

At this phase, the investigators' main goals are to demonstrate the effectiveness of a drug and to help determine possible side effects and the overall safety of the drug. Phase 2 Clinical Trials usually involve a well-designed, controlled trial in which investigators randomly select a different group of patients to receive the drug or a placebo. This phase usually *involves several hundred patients who may or may not have the actual disease* for which the drug is being developed. The data obtained from these trials primarily demonstrates the effectiveness of a particular drug and shows a clinical benefit (for example, lowering blood pressure, blood sugar, or cholesterol).

These trials will once again help to determine possible side effects and overall safety of the drug. The major drawback of these studies is the small number of patients who are being tested, which is one of the main reasons the next step, Phase 3 Clinical Trials, has become the "golden standard" for the FDA over the years.

Phase 3 Clinical Trials

In this final stage, the investigators' main goal is to further prove an experimental drug's effectiveness and safety. The FDA has the authority to stop a clinical trial if it becomes concerned about the safety of the drug, its effectiveness, or even the design of the study. Therefore it has meticulously designed Phase 3 trials to involve *several hundred to several thousand patients*. The results from these trials may provide large enough numbers to extrapolate the effectiveness and safety of the drug to the general population.

Though carefully and thoroughly administered, these clinical trials simply cannot provide the FDA, or anyone for that matter, with a true picture of all the potential side effects or dangers of new drugs once they are released to the general public. Researchers never anticipate that clinical trials reveal *all* the potential side effects and dangers of a new drug. But do you—the general public?

New Drug Application Review

Then the FDA takes the manufacturer's NDA through its review process, assigning it to a review panel made up of experts from the FDA and the medical community. Pharmacists, physicians, statisticians, and chemists—and possibly some full-time employees of the FDA or outside experts—make up the panel.

The entire review process can take from a few months to more than seven years to complete. The average length of time for approval—from the NDA to actual Approval Letter—before 1992 was approximately twenty-three months.[15] Traditionally, the FDA had been the most difficult board *in the world* through which to get a drug approved.

———

No one realizes the nature and risk of drugs more than the FDA. It knows that what may heal one person can cause a serious problem for another. But as the turn of the century drew near, memories of the Thalidomide Tragedy faded, and the FDA's determination to keep a slow and precautious attitude of approving drugs began to wear thin. An urgent tension was building, and soon the FDA would be placed under unspeakable political pressure to make the drug-approval process prompt and less arduous.

CHAPTER THREE

A Deadly Partnership

THE YEAR WAS 1990, AND WE STEPPED UP TO THE EDGE OF A new millennium wondering what promising new medical advances were in store. Thirty years had passed, and visions of the Thalidomide Tragedy had faded. The FDA remained the golden standard of protective agencies in the heart of the American consumer.

Life on the FDA's home front continued to clip along at a snail's pace, and our protector was as stubborn as ever about approving drugs according to its strict set of guidelines. The Thalidomide Tragedy was just one case in which being slow to approve a drug saved U.S. citizens tremendous sorrow. Who knows how many other dangers the FDA's persistent presence in clinical trials had quietly prevented? Though the FDA required tremendous amounts of effort, time, and money from pharmaceutical companies to get new drugs approved, we trusted the system. In fact, only a few minor legislative changes were made since the Kefauver-Harris Drug Amendments in 1962.

Until the early 1990s most drugs had been sanctioned for use in other countries long before—years before—they were considered for release in America. We couldn't have asked for a better situation in regard to the safety of the drugs in our nation. But not everyone shared these sentiments. Many Americans were chomping at the bit, ready to attack the lengthy process needed for a drug's approval in our country. The loudest voice came from U.S. citizens who were suffering from serious and fatal illnesses. Drugs that could potentially help them were available in other parts of the world, but not in the United States. People suffering from new life-threatening diseases could not wait through twenty-three months of trials for a drug to be released. Many were dying.

The AIDS epidemic became indisputable. The cry of AIDS patients had to be not only heard, but understood. People were dying horrible, painful deaths with essentially no drugs available to help them. Their lives depended on finding a cure, and time was of the essence. Never before had our nation experienced such a desperate need for speed in the approval process.

The media widely broadcast scenes of gay people and their loved ones, as well as many health-care professionals, fighting for the rights of AIDS patients. Meanwhile thousands of others suffered quietly, waiting, writing their congressmen and -women, doing all they could to relieve the pain, knowing their approaching deaths would surely arrive before the needed drugs' approval by the FDA. The rapid spread of life-threatening diseases was quickly outdating the tightfisted, time-consuming control of our great protector, or so it seemed.

Jeremy's Story

When I first held Jeremy, his head cradled perfectly in my palm and his toes barely reached the crook of my arm. I marveled at his perfect newborn body as I watched his chest rise and fall with each tiny breath. Jeremy was born in the summer heat of 1974. How relieved his mother was when his birth brought that pregnancy finally to a close!

I was the family's physician, and so Jeremy's brother and sister visited me too. Once I had to extract a bean from a nostril, and one year a fever broke out, leaving them all peppered with itchy chicken pox. I watched as each child sprouted up, and I looked forward to their visits for inoculation shots.

Jeremy Watson grew into a handsome little fella who'd come bounding into my office looking for his favorite blue chair and a *Highlights* magazine. You can imagine my concern the day Jeremy's dad carried him in with a blood-soaked towel. What first appeared to be a serious accident requiring stitches turned out to be a minor cut on his knee.

I soon diagnosed my little patient's uncontrolled bleeding as hemophilia, a congenital (genetic) disorder that usually affects males. Like his grandfather, Jeremy was unable to produce Factor VIII, which is critical in the process of clotting blood. Jeremy's parents were deeply saddened but determined to do whatever was necessary to help their son live a full life. It wasn't an easy journey, however. Because my young patient experienced significant bleeding into his soft tissues, muscles, and weight-bearing joints, he had to be treated frequently with blood products that were enriched with Factor VII in order to survive. This involved several short-term hospital stays so he could receive necessary transfusions.

One day, the specialist who was also involved in Jeremy's care called the Watson home. "I need to speak with Mrs. Watson, mother of Jeremy Watson, please."

"Speaking. How may I help you?"

"Mrs. Watson, this is Dr. Banks from the medical center. I don't want to cause you undue alarm, but we've become concerned for Jeremy regarding the blood products he's received over the past several years. Are you familiar with the new HIV virus?"

Pause. With voice shaking, she answered, "Yes."

"Mrs. Watson, none of the blood or blood products given to patients during the early 1980s was tested for this HIV virus, but we now have reason to believe it can be transmitted through blood transfusions."

Choking sobs came through the phone.

"Mrs. Watson, we need Jeremy to come in for testing."

The AIDS epidemic became known in the early 1980s, but the true cause was not fully identified until the middle of the decade. Unknowingly, many hemophiliacs across our nation were infected and developed AIDS. Jeremy was one of them; he tested positive in 1986. His parents were strong Christians, and while the homosexual crowd was protesting, Jeremy's family was praying.

Jeremy had grown into an outstanding student with a sharp mind. He's one of the few children I ever met who knew what he wanted to be when he grew up—a biochemist. Though his body had been frail most of his life, his mind was sharp and he had a photographic memory. He memorized outstanding classical piano pieces as well as the entire Gospel of Mark. At age nine he was working on a musical composition to orchestrate with the liturgy of Psalm 139. He worked hours in secret, hoping to present it to the senior pastor and his wife on their fortieth anniversary as a surprise gift.

In the meantime, fear gripped America. Was AIDS another "Black Plague"? Shouldn't AIDS patients be quarantined? Sermons, radio shows, TV programs, and magazine articles grossly misreported information about the rampant new disease. Jeremy's parents determined to allow their son to dream, as they fought quietly to protect him from ostracism from their community and church.

Jeremy never felt the blows of hateful stares from misinformed neighbors, church members, or schoolmates. Becoming extremely ill with AIDS, he was bedridden in private. His body couldn't fight against its invading infection, and he soon developed an unusual pneumonia called *Pneumocystis carinii,* in addition to a skin cancer called *Kaposi's sarcoma.*

The young boy's parents knew he didn't have long. In desperation, they searched for any latest developments in possible treatment for their dying son. Optimism glimmered when they learned of new drugs being tested, one of which was AZT, that could potentially relieve Jeremy's symptoms. But it was short-lived.

All hope was bitterly dashed when the Watsons discovered this new drug wasn't going to be available for another year or two. Jeremy couldn't possibly survive long enough for the FDA's projected date of release. The piano stood silent. Mrs. Watson carefully gathered her son's unfinished pages of music, now marked with tears, and tucked them away.

———————

Never has society so mishandled a disease. I was one of the first to teach AIDS education in our local schools, and I did so for ten years. I had several AIDS patients—people like you and me—whom the general public perceived as the lepers of our generation, cast out and alone. I've always made a special point of physically touching each of them. I hug these patients when they come to my office. If only I can bring some comfort and show them I'm not afraid of infection. I knew even then AIDS was a blood-borne disease, not something you could get from casual contact.

My hugs weren't enough; my hands were absolutely tied. I couldn't hold these precious men, women, and children tightly enough to keep them from dying before the FDA would approve drugs that could combat this horrible disease. I helplessly stood by Jeremy's side as my young patient died a painful death in 1987.

Pharmaceutical Companies Confront Congress

Pressure mounted, and the FDA found itself in the middle of turbulent waters. It could no longer disregard new diseases that were sweeping across our nation as never before, far outpacing any treatments available. Americans demanded answers. What would our government do to bring about needed change?

As you may know, people who are infected with the HIV virus typically do not develop any symptoms from their disease until eight to fifteen years after being infected. Many patients do not even realize they have AIDS until they become ill. In the 1980s and 1990s people were just beginning to learn what AIDS was all about—the hard way. Without any treatment, patients had a life expectancy of only eighteen to thirty months after becoming symptomatic from their HIV infection. Not only did potentially helpful drugs need approval more quickly, but research funds were necessary to find better treatments for AIDS.

Sick patients weren't the only Americans voicing their opinions; pharmaceutical companies were also frustrated with the FDA's approval process. The drug process time was (and is) extremely expensive, and it was time-consuming. As I mentioned in the last chapter, prior to 1992, on average a drug would take about twelve years from the development stage all the way through the approval process. If you then consider that in 1990 the FDA approved only six out of every ten drugs the pharmaceutical companies developed, you can understand the pharmaceuticals' concern.[1] (This is one of the main reasons the pharmaceutical industry must reinvest about one-fifth of its profits into research and development. On average, this is four times higher than other industries invest in research and development in the United States.)[2]

To protect their tremendous investment in research and development, drug companies must obtain patents on promising drugs early in the process. The life of a patent is approximately twenty to twenty-two years, and because of the long approval process for new drugs, most drugs only have seven to ten years left on their patents once the FDA finally approves them. Needless to say, the pharmaceutical industry pushed the FDA and Congress to find a way in which drugs could be approved more easily and quickly and in turn significantly lower their investment costs.

Congress responded favorably to the pressure. For the first time in nearly thirty years, it opened a debate regarding the FDA approval process and began looking for ways in which the process could be accelerated.

There was one insurmountable problem, however. With the pressure from the pharaceutical companies to expedite the process—as well as a genuine desire by Congress to get medications to sick people who might benefit from them faster—the FDA could not possibly fund the resources (finances and personnel) necessary to get these drugs approved any faster. This problem was made even worse by the onslaught of new drug applications they were receiving. Facing these new demands, the FDA came up stringently underfunded and understaffed.[3]

The Prescription Drug User Fee Act of 1992

In answer to the impassioned pleas of the American people and the FDA's strong urging, Congress passed the Prescription Drug User Fee Act (PDUFA) in 1992, an act impacting us heavily today. This act allowed the FDA to collect a "user's fee" from pharmaceutical companies to help cover the expense of getting new drugs approved. Congress had to choose its battles carefully, and it saw this as a way to increase funding without creating a fight for more appropriation of funds for the FDA. A corner was turned, and the world of prescription medicine was forever changed.[4]

The PDUFA of 1992 was originally a short-term experiment that Congress passed with the intent of providing the FDA with additional revenue. With sufficient funds, the FDA could immediately hire more reviewers and support staff, so they could approve drugs on a more timely basis. The pharmaceutical companies directly paid up to $250,000 with each New Drug Application; Congress expected the FDA to collect more than $329 million over the following five years (the length of time the legislation covered). The agency would then be able to hire an additional seven hundred drug reviewers and support staff through the end of 1997, at which time Congress would review the legislation to determine its success and pitfalls.[5]

It looked like a win, win, win situation.

Since the introduction of "user's fees," the FDA has been successful in approving drugs much faster. In fact, Total Approval Times, the time from the initial submission of a New Drug Application to the issuance of an Approval Letter, was actually cut in half—dropping from an average of twenty-three months to twelve months. Total Approval Time for *priority* applications—"fast-tracking"—dropped from an average of twelve months to six months.[6]

PDUFA 1992 was a huge success in the minds of many people. Patients supported it because they could get access to new medications faster. Congress supported the five-year experiment because it wouldn't cost the government additional monies. The pharmaceutical industry was excited because the cost of user's fees to a company was nothing compared to the cost of delays in the approval process the FDA created. Even the FDA was happy, because it finally received the help it needed to do its job faster and more efficiently.

Still, a murmur of disconcerted voices began to rumble and steadily grow louder. Not everyone was comfortable with the long-term consequences that were sure to result from PDUFA's success in speeding up drug reviews.

"It's a terrible system," claimed Sidney Wolfe, M.D., director of Public Citizens' Health Research Group in Washington, D.C. "The review of new drugs is too important to leave to 'user fees'." In Wolfe's opinion, the drug industry's financial support for FDA's review system was like charging criminals "user fees" to pay for the police department.[7]

> In Wolfe's opinion, the drug industry's financial support for FDA's review system was like charging criminals "user fees" to pay for the police department.

Wolfe was not the only naysayer. Other critics made public their concern that making the FDA dependent on pharmaceutical company funding diminished the agency's independence and objectivity. Basically, these critics believed that with the passing of PDUFA, the FDA landed in the pharmaceutical industry's pocket. Wolfe's group argued before Congress that funding the FDA's drug reviews with pharmaceutical money "lowered U.S. drug safety standards, arguably once considered the best in the world."[8]

I couldn't agree more.

PDUFA answered the desperate cries of the dying . . . but not without a cost—a great cost indeed. PDUFA was the handshake that created what I call the "deadly partnership."

The Deadly Partnership

Congress had formed a partnership between the FDA and the pharmaceutical companies, and our "great protector" would now receive a significant amount of its funding from the industry it was intended to regulate. This legislation would also require the Food and Drug Administration not only to work closely with pharmaceutical companies in getting their drugs approved, but also to get their drugs approved in a significantly shorter time.

Since the approval process itself is such a significant factor for the drug industry's research and development costs, Congress was willing to oblige pharmaceutical companies in their demands. As a result, the percentage of funding for the FDA that comes from "user fees" is approaching 50 percent of the FDA's total budget.[9]

With the new partnership came an undeniable shift for the FDA. Unfortunately, Congress had not foreseen that the new legislation would distort the distribution of labor at the FDA. By becoming primarily focused on fast-tracking new drugs, the agency had to short-change other vital functions that protect the public, such as post-marketing surveillance of serious adverse drug reactions. The departments that worked on the post-marketing surveillance were responsible for identifying additional adverse drug reactions after drugs had been released by the FDA for use by the general public. With the great internal shifts in the FDA toward drug approval, surveillance departments began consistently receiving relatively less and less funding.[10]

This was an ideal scenario for the pharmaceutical industry. For them, the new partnership was working out nicely. Because the FDA now had to meet certain performance goals, it was approving 80 percent of all new drug applications (compared to the 60 percent it approved prior to PDUFA).[11] Now that the FDA was sanctioning drugs much *more quickly,* this allowed companies to launch *more new drugs*, in *half the time* to the public. And due to lack of funds and staffing in the postmarketing surveillance department, the agency was slow to recognize any serious adverse side effects after it approved the drug. A manufacturer's product most likely would remain on the market much longer, regardless of ill effects it had on people.

The Food and Drug Administration Modernization Act of 1997

PDUFA appeared to be a success, but not only did the drug-approval process need more funds, it definitely still needed further improvement.

Five years had passed, and the time had come for its review. What was going to happen to the partnership? What would happen if Congress didn't renew the legislation? Money did the talking.

Congress and the FDA were aware of the seriousness of existing problems and set out to correct them through the Food and Drug Administration Modernization Act of 1997 (FDAMA). PDUFA put a turbo boost on drug approval, but this new legislation would represent the most sweeping changes in FDA functions since 1938. It not only extended user's fees for an additional five years, it also opened several floodgates in drug approval. The deadly partnership continued.

FDAMA 1997 included three amendments that brought profound and lasting implications to the pharmaceutical industry: "off-label" use of drugs; drug labeling for children; and fast-tracking (accelerated) approval. On the surface these changes appeared to be a positive advancement in medicine, but an opposite reality also became true. The amendments monumentally increased the margin for patients' developing adverse drug reactions.

Following is a detailed explanation of each amendment.

"Off-Label" Use of Drugs

Congress and the FDA knew physicians were using many prescription medications for situations and diseases for which the FDA never approved. This was entirely legal. But up until this point, the FDA had prohibited pharmaceutical companies from promoting alternative uses of their medications directly to physicians. Prior to 1997, pharmaceutical reps were never allowed to promote a drug for a treatment other than its prescribed use.[12]

The new legislation did away with the longstanding prohibition of giving out information on unapproved uses of drugs by the manufacturer. Drug companies now had permission to circulate information on the use of their drug for diseases or clinical situations that the FDA had never approved. Reps could suggest the sale of new drugs for uses with no proof of safety or effectiveness, such as a seizure drug that could also be used as a painkiller.

Pharmaceutical companies had won again. Their reps now frequently share alternative uses of their drugs in my office, even though the success and safety of these alternative uses have never been formally established.[13] (The only stipulation currently pending for pharmaceutical companies is they must file a supplemental application to the FDA within three years, as well as provide appropriate research to establish the safety and efficacy of the off-label drug for the unapproved use.)

Drug Labeling for Children

Adults purchase most new drugs. Therefore, drug companies usually do not conduct additional clinical studies to determine dosages and safety in children. As a result, there has been a growing trend of using adult drugs (clinical trial done on adults only) for treatment of children.

With the FDAMA legislation, Congress attempted to address this problem. According to Donna Schuster, M.D., of the American Academy of Pediatrics, physicians "prescribe drugs for children based on information from limited medical studies, clinical experience and simple observation." Although this is entirely legal, said Schuster, "clinical trials in children would provide more precise information, so that exact dosages could be determined."[14]

When drug labels do not include adequate pediatric information, health-care providers use what they have available, often being forced to play a guessing game about dosage amounts that may compromise the care of the patient. This is no small problem in the United States. Duane Alexander, M.D., director of the National Institute of Child Health and Human Development, stated in 1998 that "three-quarters of medications on the U.S. market today are not labeled for use in children."[15] And this fact is still true today.

Many children died using the drug Propulsid.[16] Doctors knew that it was effective in adults but did not have any data on dosages and safety in infants and children. Pediatricians presumed the drug to be safe after its approval for use in adults. (See Chapter 6.)

For years the FDA had realized this shortcoming and finally

attempted to address the problem in this particular legislation. With the ruling of FDAMA, the FDA can now require drug companies to conduct additional clinical trials to provide prescribing information specifically for children. In exchange, the drug company receives an additional six months on its drug's patent.[17]

This may help physicians with future drugs and even some recently released drugs. But the new ruling doesn't go far enough. Pharmaceutical companies still have little incentive to look at drugs that are already off patent. When drugs are "off patent," the brand-name drug is no longer protected by a patent, leading to the development of generic drugs. Though FDAMA made great strides toward future drug labeling for children, we still have an overwhelming problem.

> Only five of the eighty most frequently used drugs in newborns and infants have pediatric use instructions—meaning only 5 percent have been tested in pediatric clinical trials!

According to Dr. Alexander, only five of the eighty most frequently used drugs in newborns and infants have pediatric use instructions—meaning only 5 percent have been tested in pediatric clinical trials![18]

Accelerated Approval and Parallel Tracking

Prior to 1992, the FDA had always had the reputation of being stringent and unrelenting in its standards. It had long been the FDA's position that to achieve "substantial evidence" (in other words, standard proof of a drug's effectiveness), it must require at least *two* "well-controlled" Phase 3 Clinical Trials. Another noticeable shift brought about by FDAMA 1997 is the agency's willingness to approve a drug based on a single study.[19] (The FDA holds that two well-done clinical trials will still be the standard, but it will accept a single study in some situations.)

Among other provisions FDAMA made, the Food and Drug Administration must now consider early approval of drugs that address unmet needs resulting from serious or life-threatening conditions. Furthermore, the agency will help speed availability of experimental drugs to patients using what is called "parallel tracking." Under this policy, patients with such life-threatening diseases as AIDS or cancer, whose condition prevents them from participating in controlled clinical trials, can receive investigational drugs that are showing early potential benefits. For example, a terminally ill patient who is too sick to actually participate in a drug study can still receive an experimental drug that can potentially help him or her.[20]

Quicker Drug Approval—But What About Safety?

PDUFA and FDAMA brought about definite improvement in the speed with which the FDA now approves drugs. The Food and Drug Administration has indeed accomplished its goals in meeting proposed deadlines, and the pharmaceutical industry seems satisfied to have supplemental funds coming in.[21]

We cannot deny that the accelerated process of the FDA and availability of new drugs have extended the lives of thousands of patients desperate for these new drugs. And it has certainly bolstered America's economy in the pharmaceutical industry! We must acknowledge, however, the dramatic role reversal of the FDA and wonder what this means for our nation's safety.

Once believed to be the major watchdog and protector of its people, the FDA is no longer an objective overseer. I don't know about you, but I don't believe the FDA should be friends with anyone. The agency's duty is to remain independent from all outside influences—without conflict of interest. After all, its job is to regulate the pharmaceutical companies and the drugs they produce.

Many in our nation are losing faith in the quality of the FDA's drug-approval process. The agency's true heart and the effectiveness of the latest drug approval system need to be seriously scrutinized. Where the agency once had a tough attitude and didn't let anything slip by, it has found itself in a precariously cooperative role with the pharmaceutical industry. The question is no longer, "*Should* this drug be approved?" but instead, "*How* can we get this drug approved?"

CHAPTER FOUR

The Great Clinical Trial—You!

MEET ALICE. WITH EYES BRIGHT, SHE REMEMBERS HOW PEOPLE exclaimed at her fiftieth wedding anniversary that she didn't look a day over sixty. Now in her fifty-third year of marriage to Frank, her husband is not the only one who finds Alice beautiful. With smooth, firm skin and a pleasant figure, she often receives compliments on how young she looks.

One would hardly guess by looking that Alice is a seventy-four-year-old grandmother with ten grandchildren. At each year of age, Alice tells her children, "This is the best year of my life." And each year truly has been. In good health, Alice had found her only persistent problem to be a spastic colon, or what I call irritable bowel syndrome.

She had been taking Lomotil or sometimes Immodium AD to control her symptoms, but neither drug worked very well. Her bowel problem was more of a nuisance than anything serious. But after she had had four different GI workups, her doctor assured her that irritable bowel syndrome was the diagnosis, and it was something she would have to live with.

During Linda's annual checkup, she mentioned that she was still having a considerable amount of trouble with her bowels in spite of using the medication prescribed. Her doctor's eyes lit up, and he told her there was a new drug that the FDA had just released that would correct her problem. He had prescribed it for several of his patients, and they were having great results. The drug was called Lotronex. It was the first new drug to be released for irritable bowel syndrome in years. You can understand how anxious she was to try it.

Alice was delighted with the results of the new drug. She no longer suffered from diarrhea, cramping, or bloating. She could go to restaurants or have dinner with friends and not be embarrassed by having to excuse herself to run to the bathroom. Delighted, Alice began telling her friends how wonderful this new medication was.

A month passed, and one day Alice noticed she had not had a bowel movement for at least two days. She was eating normally but had no urge to use the restroom. Two days later, still no movement. She started feeling discomfort from significant bloating in her abdomen, and soon she felt increasing abdominal pain.

Frank grew worried and took her to the local emergency room for an evaluation. The ER physician was noticeably concerned and ordered blood work and x-ray films of her abdomen. The x-rays showed major distention of her entire colon. Her white blood cell count was also sky-high. He quickly called in a local general surgeon.

After the general surgeon evaluated Alice, he recommended an immediate operation and possible resection of part or all of her colon. Frank and Alice agreed to the surgery because they both realized how serious the situation had become. The general surgeon found that her colon was almost black due to a lack of blood supply. He had no other choice than to remove her entire colon. This meant that she would need an ileostomy or a stoma, where the small bowel would be open to the surface of the abdomen. Alice would use a bag the rest of her life.

Alice did recover nicely, and her pain and fever improved over the next few days. The surgeon informed Alice and Frank that this was truly a rare occurrence of ischemic colitis. He said that because the entire colon had lost its blood supply, it had actually died. There was nothing he could do to save it. He believed the new drug Lotronex had been the culprit. Alice would live the rest of her life with the ileostomy. She considers herself extremely lucky to be alive.

The FDA took Lotronex off the market several months later because so many patients had similar problems to Alice's with ischemic colitis. But unlike her, many patients actually died. After reading the reports on the FDA's decision to remove the drug from the marketplace, Frank and Alice were puzzled to learn that FDA had given it fast-track status—meaning the FDA had approved Lotronex rapidly. They were baffled when everything they read indicated fast-track status was supposed to be reserved for lifesaving drugs or new therapies for serious diseases.

Irritable bowel syndrome is anything *but* a serious disease. Alice said that it was a major inconvenience for her, but definitely nothing critical. Of even more concern was the fact that the premarketing trials of Lotronex reported cases of ischemic colitis and severe constipation. The FDA had decided to release the drug anyway. The drug was on the market for only ten months before it had to be removed.

Unknowingly, Alice had become part of the great clinical trial.

Troubles on the Fast Track for Lotronex

In 1999, the FDA agreed to place Lotronex, a medication to treat irritable bowel syndrome, on the fast track for drug approval. Irritable bowel is a functional problem of the gastrointestinal tract that leads to bloating, cramping, and either constipation or diarrhea. It is not, however, a serious medical condition and rarely leads to hospitalization.

During its premarket clinical trials, an FDA official noted four cases of ischemic colitis (when the bowels do not receive enough blood supply), which is a real problem and can even be life-threatening.

During the clinical trials 27 percent of the patients who took Lotronex developed significant constipation, compared to only 5 percent in the control group, which had taken a placebo. This brought definite concern, because it was a drug given primarily for symptomatic relief of a benign disease.

Though some FDA reviewers believed Lotronex "was capable" of causing potentially life-threatening complications, the pharmaceutical company's seeming lack of concern regarding the assessment of the risk of ischemic colitis swayed the advisory committee, which approved the drug on February 9, 2000.

It was not long after Lotronex was on the market that a stream of voluntary reports poured into the FDA relating Lotronex with numerous cases of ischemic colitis. More than ninety hospital admissions for severe constipation were also reported in patients taking the new drug. Several of these patients required surgery, and some needed to have their entire colons removed. The FDA withdrew the drug on November 28, 2000.[1]

The Great Clinical Trial

If you remember nothing else, remember this: fewer than 50 percent of all of the serious adverse reactions to a new drug the FDA releases are identified prior to its release into the marketplace.[2] That is correct: half of the damaging side effects are yet to be discovered after a drug is released onto the market! How does the FDA find out about the other 50 percent of the serious side effects of a new drug? The answer is quite simple: it relies on *you*.

You are the most important "clinical trial" when it comes to truly finding *all* of the serious adverse effects of a drug. Phase 3 Clinical Trials (see Chapter 2) usually involve only a few hundred to a few thousand people whom the drug company recruits. The small number of patients involved in these trials allows the FDA to identify merely the most *common*—not necessarily the most *serious*—side effects that a particular drug may have.[3]

It is important to remember that the FDA conducts premarketing clinical trials with patients who are either very healthy or who have *only* the disease for which the drug is being tested. *Why?* Drug companies

can fund the research of only a limited number of patients in the preclinical trials. A drug company couldn't possibly afford to pay for clinical trials that involve the tens of thousands of patients needed to make
these drugs safer by determining *all* the adverse drug reactions. Instead,
they rely on postmarketing surveillance.

Though we can appreciate the need for speed while approving new
drugs to treat life-threatening diseases, we are left to marvel at the
power granted the FDA in pushing drugs through the approval process
for conditions such as irritable bowel syndrome. The last legislation,
FDAMA, trimmed months, and in some cases years, from a drug's
inception to the moment it's put into the hands of the consumer. We
wonder why drugs such as Lotronex are being granted fast-track status.
What's the urgency?

Let's say I am a drug company that is trying to develop a new and
effective high blood pressure medication. I'll be spending close to half
a billion dollars in research and development, so it is only logical that I
want these preclinical studies to succeed! So wouldn't I do everything
within my power and control to be sure that this drug is eventually
approved by the FDA? My main focus is getting the FDA's approval of
the new drug as quickly and as inexpensively as possible. Wouldn't I
then recruit individuals into my study group who *only* have high blood
pressure and who are otherwise very healthy? This would give me the
best chance to decrease any potential adverse drug reactions during
these preclinical trials, and have my drug approved by the FDA. It is
beneficial for me to have both a safe and effective drug. However, with
this amount of money at risk, wouldn't it seem logical that I would
want everything, as much as humanly possible, to be in my favor?

I know that once my drug is released to the general public, patients
who are in much poorer health (those who are typically taking several
different medications at the same time) will begin taking the new drug,
and this is when the majority of the serious adverse drug reactions will
be discovered. Other reactions will become apparent only after the drug
has been used for a couple of years, and identifying these reactions will
truly be difficult. This is the case for all medication. There is no way the

preclinical trials are able to determine *all* the serious adverse drug reactions. As a pharmaceutical company, it is my hope that there will be only minor adverse drug reactions discovered after the drug is released. However, this is unknown territory, and only time will truly tell.

Thank You, General Public!

Tremendous marketing strategies accompany the release of a drug to the public when the FDA approves it. According to the *New York Times*, sales forces of the largest forty drug companies in the U.S. "exploded" in recent years. In 1994, pharmaceutical companies employed 35,000 full-time representatives to visit doctors and "detail" them on their companies' drugs. By 1998, that number had grown to 56,000, averaging one salesperson for every eleven physicians. Drug companies actually spent $6.3 billion in the first eleven months of 1998 marketing their products directly to physicians. These same companies spent nearly $2 billion in 1999 marketing their drugs directly to you—the patient.[4]

Don't you just love being interrupted by prescription medication commercials while watching your favorite TV program? "Life is good; troubles are now gone. No more allergies; no sign of high cholesterol." Happy people are dancing through flower fields or standing at the edge of a rock precipice with their hair blowing in the wind. "This drug will forever change your life . . ." Then in turbo speed a voice runs through all the known possible risks involved. I'm sure it's never occurred to you these are only half of the possible symptoms that could arise with that particular drug. If the rest were known, they would have to list those too, but then you'd never get back to your program.

Many of us don't find the amount of money spent on marketing *prescription drugs to physicians* surprising, but when considering the billions of dollars spent on marketing *prescription drugs to the public*, don't you wonder why? After all, you can obtain prescription*s* only through a doctor. Pharmaceutical companies are willing to spend this kind of advertising money on only their most recently approved medication. Why? Could it be that they are in the business of making money?

Surveys reported in our medical literature reveal that when a patient comes into a doctor's office and requests a specific drug that he has seen advertised in the media, the doctor writes *the exact prescription the patient requested* more than 70 percent of the time![5] No wonder we hardly watch a favorite TV program, or read the newspaper or a magazine without seeing advertisements for prescription medications.

"I want to try the new 'purple pill'," my patients will say, "the one I saw on TV." Or maybe they'll ask for one of the most recent arthritis medications. Every day I am reminded that pharmaceutical marketing campaigns are a huge success.

> "Voluntary" here means that when a physician or other medical professional suspects that a drug has caused a serious adverse drug reaction, he or she is not required to report it to the FDA.

Have you ever wondered if you should consider taking a new drug or continue taking a newly released sample prescription? If so, you need to understand how the FDA and physicians learn (or fail to learn) about new serious adverse drug reactions once the FDA releases a drug on the open market.

Monitoring Drug Safety

The process of monitoring drug safety in the U.S. begins with our voluntary reporting system channeled through a special department in the FDA called the Office of Postmarketing Drug Risk Assessment. After a drug appears on the market, physicians can make voluntary reports of its potential adverse side effects to the pharmaceutical company and to the FDA. "Voluntary" here means that when a physician or other medical professional suspects that a drug has caused a serious adverse drug reaction, he or she is *not* required to report it to the FDA.[6] It is estimated that less than 1 percent of all the adverse drug reactions are actually being reported to the FDA.[7] This is a pivotal point in determining our safety.

For instance, if Alice's physician were one of the less than 1 percent who took the time to research her case, fill out complicated forms, and submit the report of her severe reaction to the FDA, the Office of

Postmarketing Drug Risk Assessment would receive the report. There, approximately two-thirds of the staff is assigned to data entry, verification, or review of such data. Once the staff identifies a possible serious problem with a drug, such as the life-threatening side effect of ischemic colitis from Lotronex, it has little authority or power other than reporting its findings back to the advisory committee *that originally approved the drug.* [8]

This advisory committee may take some sort of action, question the findings, or ask for additional information. But once a new serious adverse drug reaction (ADR) is identified beyond doubt, the most common action for an advisory committee is to change the product label (or "package insert"). If this new drug reaction is especially serious, the FDA will send out a "Dear Doctor" letter to every physician in the country, warning him of the new label change in the drug's package insert. [9]

If an acute problem occurs that went unrecognized during the approval process, the committee may even decide to create a "black box" warning in the package insert. This "black box" warning is just that—a bold, printed warning about the potential adverse drug reaction surrounded by a black box.

Black Box Warning for SELDANE

QTc Interval prolongation/ventricular arrhythmia rare cases of serious cardiovascular adverse events, including death, cardiac arrest, torsades de pointes, and other ventricular arrhythmias, have been observed in the following clinical settings, frequently in association with increased terfenadine levels which lead to electro-cardiographic QTc prolongation:

1. Concomitant administration of Ketoconazole (Nizoral) or Itraconazole (Sporanox)
2. Overdose, including single Terfenadine doses as low as 360 mg.
3. Concomitant administration of Clarithromycin, Erythromycin, or Troleadomycin
4. Significant Hepatic Dysfunction

Terfenadine is contraindicated in patients taking Ketoconazole, Itraconazole, Erythromycin, Clarithromycin, or Troleadomycin, and in patients with significant hepatic dysfunction.

Do not exceed recommended dose.

In some cases, severe arrhythmias have been preceded by episodes of syncope. Syncope in patients receiving Terfenadine should lead to discontinuation of treatment and full evaluation of potential arrhythmias.

Alice may have felt a sense of relief (albeit a minor one) knowing that, because of the voluntary report her doctor made in follow-up to her adverse reaction, perhaps others could avoid suffering altogether. In the case of Lotronex, voluntary reports played an important role in having the drug pulled from the market. However, most of the time these reports result only in a mere label change.

The advisory committee responsible for a particular drug's approval may not be able to determine whether the evidence from a pre-marketing clinical trial or reports of a particular adverse drug reaction point to a true problem or not. Not everything is black and white when it comes to dealing with potential adverse drug reactions. Sometimes the Food and Drug Administration needs more data to make a definitive determination about a particular ADR.

> The FDA must rely on the drug company to provide the data on deaths and illnesses caused *by the company's own products.*

Due to its limitation of funds, the FDA may require a drug company to perform postmarket trials on a specific drug with suspected ADRs. Congress has specifically restricted any of the funds received from "user fees" to be used for monitoring drug safety.[10] This will determine if the drug indeed may have a problem. As a result, the FDA must rely on the drug company to provide the data on deaths and illnesses caused *by the company's own products.*

Does this raise any red flags in your mind? Why would a pharmaceutical company be excited about performing these studies? The FDA would then possibly have information needed to pull the pharmaceutical's drug off the market. It should come as no surprise, then, that the FDA has never withdrawn a drug from the market based on postmarket clinical trials that a drug company performed.[11]

So how does the FDA actually withdraw a drug from the marketplace? As you can see from this discussion, this is not a common action. The FDA typically requires a long, arduous process before it will withdraw a drug once the agency has approved it. The evidence against a particular drug has to be overwhelming, and even then it may not be enough most of the time.

Prescription Drugs Under Investigation

The Federal Aviation Administration (FAA) establishes the standards by which airplanes are built, licensed, and flown. But when a plane crashes, a *different organization, independent of the FAA*, steps in to investigate the crash. This agency is known as the National Transportation Safety Board (NTSB). Why? The intrinsic need for objectivity demands nothing less. This board was established because a second independent agency was needed to eliminate any conflict of interest within the FAA while investigating crashes of planes it had approved and licensed.

This is not the case, however, with the FDA. In fact, not only does the same agency conduct the investigations, as I have mentioned, the same individuals who approved the drug *lead* the investigations. FDA officials involved in the new drug-approval process may spend up to a year of their lives evaluating a drug before approving it for release on the market. Therefore, I find it highly unlikely that those same individuals who were involved in recommending the drug for approval would later conduct a dispassionate evaluation of possible harm the drug may be causing. Don't you think the most likely reaction would be to defend

> The FDA removes a drug from the market only when the evidence is so overwhelming and the pressure so great that the organization has no other choice.

their earlier decision—especially if there were early warning signs during the preclinical trials that a drug could cause this particular drug reaction?

As I've mentioned, following their evaluation, the original committee may then take several courses of action. It might question the findings or ask for additional information. If this is a new and previously unrecognized drug reaction, however, 99 percent of the time it will require only a label change. The FDA rarely takes a drug off the market. Remember this: the FDA removes a drug from the market only when the evidence is so overwhelming and the pressure so great that the organization has no other choice.[12]

American Guinea Pigs

Whether we know it or not, Americans are now the subjects used to determine the safety of some of the most dangerous drugs in the world. If you have purchased newly released drugs or have taken free samples of medication, you, too, are part of the great ongoing clinical trial.

Another alarming fact is most of the medications that reached our shores before 1992 had already been tested and used by millions of patients in various countries throughout the world, which means the most dangerous ones were removed from the market before they ever had a chance to be released in the United States. That, my friend, is no longer the case.

Before 1990, only 3 to 4 percent of all new drugs were first released in the United States. Now, 66 percent of all new drugs being released in the world today are being approved and released *first* in the United States.[13] Citizens of America have unknowingly become the guinea pigs for the majority of new drugs released into the world today. Coupled with the difficulty of having a drug removed once it is considered dangerous, we should be shocked and even outraged.

> Before 1990, only 3 to 4 percent of all new drugs were first released in the United States. Now, 66 percent of all new drugs being released in the world today are being approved and released first in the United States.

Are you a participating subject in the "great clinical trial"? Americans must realize that the main focus of the Food and Drug Administration has shifted to getting new drugs approved, not ensuring their safety. In an article published in the May 1, 2002, issue of the *Journal of the American Medical Association,* Dr. Karen Lasser supported this argument. She wrote, "Prior to approval, drugs are studied in selected populations for limited periods, possibly contributing to an increased risk of adverse drug reactions after approval." In addition, she confirmed that "pharmaceutical companies frequently market drugs heavily to both patients and clinicians before the full range of adverse drug reactions (ADRs) is ascertained." [14]

While the FDA is approving drugs at an unprecedented rate, resources for postmarketing drug surveillance remain significantly lacking. We can no longer disregard the potentially far-reaching damage wrought when we consider the unknown danger of new drugs coupled with the rush of competing interests during development and marketing.

————

The next time you see a new prescription commercial, make a mental note that at the end of the commercial they are listing only the most common side-effects. Less than half the side-effects are even known at that time. Also keep in mind that as result of having only a voluntary reporting system in place, no one truly knows how frequently a particular drug reaction may be occurring. Remember that the FDA accepts most serious adverse drug reactions as the inherent risk of taking any medication. Our protector will make claims that the system works, and if you are one of the survivors, it has worked for you. If only one hundred thousand others this year could be so fortunate.

PART II

SYSTEM GONE WRONG

CHAPTER FIVE

The Rezulin Story

DO YOU REMEMBER THE MOVIE *THE FUGITIVE*, STARRING Harrison Ford as Dr. Richard Kimble? In the movie, Kimble, a well-respected vascular surgeon, is wrongfully accused and convicted of murdering his wife. While guards are transferring him to the penitentiary, Kimble has a turn of fate and makes a narrow escape from a tangle of grinding metal after the penitentiary bus collides with an oncoming freight train. He is free to find the real killer.

The chase is on! U.S. Marshall Sam Gerard (Tommy Lee Jones) begins his relentless pursuit. Tension mounts as Kimble wriggles out of several near-captures. Flashbacks of his beautiful wife, brutally killed by a one-armed assassin, tear through the fugitive's memory as he tries to piece together the motive of the murder. Do you remember what it was? While keeping his identity hidden, Dr. Kimble unravels the mystery alone.

Pieces start coming together as Kimble recalls an onslaught of patients with unusual symptoms. These patients were suffering from bleeding problems related to liver damage. All participants of a clinical trial sponsored by Chicago Memorial Hospital, these patients experienced bleeding as a result of taking an experimental drug called RDU90 (Provasic).

In the movie, sales of the new drug Provasic had topped $7.5 billion in its first year, and its manufacturer was promoting it as having absolutely no side effects. Having unearthed a major cover-up of the severe adverse drug reactions Provasic did indeed cause, Dr. Kimble was now an undeniable threat to its market. As the story progresses, the truth is finally revealed: the pharmaceutical company hired a one-armed hit man to take out Kimble. The doctor had been the target all along.

———

Significantly overdramatized, *The Fugitive* brought to life the multibillion-dollar industry of pharmaceuticals and the politics often involved in producing and marketing a new drug—though I hardly believe pharmaceutical companies hire hit men to remove any potential threats. Still, as you learn about the diabetes drug, Rezulin, you will recognize new aspects of what I explained in Chapter 3 as a "deadly partnership."

You Picked a Winner!

The large corporation Warner-Lambert has placed some of America's finest products, from Listerine mouthwash to Halls cough drops, on the market. In fact, its pharmaceutical division performed so well in the early nineties, they boasted company sales of $7 billion a year![1]

When Warner-Lambert's top seller, the cholesterol pill Lopid, went off patent, the company's sales began to dive. Still, the company showed little concern. It was confident the newly approved Alzheimer's medication, Cognex, would pull it through its financial slump with its promising sales potential. Unfortunately, the drug did not perform as well as Warner-Lambert had hoped, and it did not regain its much-needed profit margin.

Scrambling for a recovery in sales, compromises were made, and by November of 1995 *Warner-Lambert pleaded guilty to a felony of concealing deficiencies from the FDA* in its manufacturing of several other drugs.[2] Lack of integrity is disturbing news, but in the world of business, progress marches on. Warner-Lambert agreed to pay a $10 million fine (one of the largest ever imposed on a pharmaceutical company), and all was forgiven.[3] The company committed anew to push forward in the development of a new, profitable medication.

Just four months later, Warner-Lambert proudly announced its successful comeback by highlighting a new breakthrough drug for diabetes called Rezulin. The pharmaceutical company claimed that once approved, this drug would become one of the largest-selling medications the company had ever marketed.

Its new drug Rezulin offered the best hope of putting a new winner on its team. It was the first truly new diabetic medication to be introduced in over twenty years. Even more exciting was the fact that this drug actually attacked the root cause of over 90 percent of the diabetics in the United States—insulin resistance. Rezulin had the potential of becoming one of the most profitable drugs ever. The quicker the company could get this drug on the market, the better for everyone—the company and the diabetic patients. The company's mission statement would be put to the test: "Every day a new product fails to reach a market means missed opportunity."[4]

> A pharmaceutical company's mission statement: "Every day a new product fails to reach a market means missed opportunity."

How does a pharmaceutical company ensure that its drug is a winner? The legislative process must be fast, smart, and persuasive. Warner-Lambert would rely heavily on its new partner, the FDA, in the race against the clock, with fast-track status. Warner-Lambert submitted a formal NDA (New Drug Application) to the Food and Drug Administration and, with no idle time afforded, it hammered out new marketing strategies while waiting for the FDA to announce its new drug was safe and effective.

Life on the Fast Track

For the first time in the history of the FDA it granted a drug fast-track status for a condition other than a life-threatening disease. Remember that the FDA was to reserve the fast-track designation only for drugs indicated for illnesses such as cancer or AIDS, not chronic diseases like diabetes. Warner-Lambert, I am sure, was not disappointed in the fact that the FDA had decided to put its new drug on the fast track.

Warner-Lambert paid its user's fee, and the FDA set to work. It assigned the job of evaluating Rezulin's safety and effectiveness, a task that would prove challenging, to Dr. John Gueriguian, a veteran FDA medical officer.

You might imagine that when a researcher finds anything other than great news for a drug—especially one on the fast track—his colleagues may not appreciate what he has to say, and Gueriguian was not the bearer of good news. After initial evaluation of the clinical trials, the medical officer discovered definite "red flags" implying potential heart and liver damage with the use of Rezulin. To make matters worse, he didn't find Rezulin to have any significant benefits over other treatments already on the market. As predicted, Gueriguian's unbiased findings were not taken kindly.[5]

According to a story in the *Los Angeles Times*, Gueriguian came under heavy fire from Warner-Lambert executives following his report. On November 4, 1996, the FDA removed John Gueriguian from the evaluation of Rezulin, with insistence that he have no further dealings with Warner-Lambert. Curiously, Dr. Gueriguian's medical review and evaluation were purged from the FDA's files as well.[6]

The Specific Concerns About Rezulin

Effects on the Heart

In spite of the treatment of Gueriguian and his evaluation, the FDA was concerned about the potential risk of heart damage with the use of Rezulin. Gueriguian's reports revealed that initial animal studies conducted on three different species showed all three developed enlarged, gray hearts in reaction to the drug.[7] This was the first time Gueriguian ever recalled all species of animals demonstrating an adverse effect.

Fulfilling its obligations, the FDA required Warner-Lambert to conduct clinical trials on humans to assess the drug's effect on human hearts.

Warner-Lambert ordered the Echo Study (see boxed information) to be done on healthy people; a follow-up study for those with preexisting heart disease; and reports to be filed for those who died due to heart failure. Though the FDA appeared to have covered all its tracks, research conclusions would eventually prove to be either flawed, disregarded, or never gathered.[8]

The Echo Study

This particular clinical trial used an echocardiogram to evaluate Rezulin's effect on the human heart.

The study used 154 healthy subjects at five different sites. The investigators performed baseline evaluations of all the patients' hearts before they administered the medication. These subjects then took Rezulin for forty-eight weeks. At the end of the term, further echocardiograms evaluated their heart functions.

The FDA showed apprehension when 26 percent of the study's subjects dropped out. With more than one-fourth of the subjects not completing the study, the results would be skewed. What conclusive evidence could they find, since so many of the participants withdrew? In spite of the time pressure, with only three weeks left before the final decision was to be made for Rezulin, the FDA sent out a pharmacist to two of the sites to survey the results directly.

The pharmacist found definite irregularities in the interpretation of the echocardiograms. At one of the sites, the echocardiograms showed a substantial increase in the left ventricular mass (meaning the heart was larger in size than it was before the patient started taking the drug).

After all was said and done, senior FDA officials concluded that the conduct of the study at these two sites was definitely "flawed," so the results were ignored.[9]

Effects on the Liver

According to Gueriguian, liver complications were also apparent in early studies on Rezulin. Although no subjects actually developed liver failure in the premarketing clinical trials of Rezulin, approximately 2 percent of the patients showed evidence of increased liver enzymes on follow-up blood tests (evidence that liver cells are dying).[10] These findings are what researchers call "soft evidence"—an indicator of potentially more serious problems once the drug is released onto the open market.

Soft evidence on Rezulin should have brought about more concern for the FDA. The drug, after all, was to be taken over a period of several years in order to reduce severe complications of diabetes such as blindness, amputation, and kidney failure. The long-term side effects should have been presented clearly and careful consideration made as to whether the side effects would indeed outweigh the benefits of the drug.

Perhaps the FDA was under great time pressure since it had granted fast-track status to Rezulin, but to my disbelief, the agency disregarded the soft evidence of increased liver enzymes and granted approval of Rezulin with *absolutely no warning* in the first package insert.

The ECHO study also did not give conclusive evidence that Rezulin did not cause any heart damage. For good measure, the administration went through the motions of entering into a *nonbinding* agreement with Warner-Lambert to perform a postmarketing study on diabetic patients who had evidence of heart failure, after the drug's release on the market. This would provide the FDA (and anyone else who might be concerned) the assurance that Rezulin was in fact safe. The study was never done.[11]

The Power of a Market Launch

In spite of research weaknesses, the FDA drug advisory panel *unanimously* recommended Rezulin for approval as a prescription drug. Warner-Lambert's stock soared to an all-time high the same day. True to its word, the FDA's fast track granted final approval of Rezulin almost exactly six months to the day after Warner-Lambert had filed the New Drug Application.[12] Warner-Lambert issued news releases touting Rezulin as the first antidiabetic drug to target insulin resistance. Advertisements appeared everywhere, including many medical and lay journals. The full-fledged marketing assault of its new drug had begun.

Even though the FDA encouraged Warner-Lambert to tone down its claims in its advertisements, Warner-Lambert still presented Rezulin to physicians as the first major breakthrough in more than twenty years for treating diabetes. Pharmaceutical reps flooded doctors' offices like mine, peddling their newly approved drug and distributing loads of free samples.

The medical community responded with excitement to the release of Rezulin. Three articles appeared in the March 26, 1998 issue of the *New England Journal of Medicine* praising the effectiveness of Rezulin. Studies reviewed by the articles' authors explained that in cases where the new drug was given alone to insulin-treated patients with Type II diabetes mellitus, significant improvement resulted, and patients were able to decrease the amount of insulin they were taking.[13, 14] Our hopes soared high.

Warner-Lambert's hopes soared high, too. Rezulin was an immediate hit! Physicians began putting millions of patients on Rezulin within months of its release. Since this was a medication that patients had to take continually over a long period of time, the pharmaceutical company's projected sales and profits were coming true.

But the quiet voice of an editorial in the *New England Journal of Medicine* gave doctors a word of caution: "Because of the possibility of drug-induced hepatic dysfunction [liver damage], therapy with Rezulin should be limited to patients who can be evaluated frequently until the incidence and severity of hepatic dysfunction with this drug become clearer."[15]

Could Rezulin Actually Prevent Diabetes?

Warner-Lambert was not satisfied with simply marketing its drug to those patients with existing diabetes. It desired to promote the new drug as having the ability to *prevent* diabetes, especially for those who were at high risk. Since insulin resistance is the underlying cause of more than 90 percent of Type II diabetes, Warner-Lambert presented Rezulin as treating *the cause* of the disease by improving the patient's sensitivity to his own insulin. In fact, potential advances of Rezulin on diabetes research were so promising that the drug was chosen as one of two drugs to be used in the prestigious, $175 million National Institute of Diabetes (NIH) study. This study involved more than three thousand volunteers with preclinical diabetes at twenty-seven different research centers around the United States to see if the drug could prevent the disease. The claim, in the company's own words: "Rezulin has the potential to virtually redefine the diabetes market open to millions of patients around the world," according to Lodewijk de Vink, president of Warner-Lambert.[16]

You can appreciate Warner-Lambert's excitement over its new drug. After all, more than 16 million Americans suffer from diabetes, and 24 million more patients have preclinical diabetes. All of these patients would be possible candidates for Rezulin. The company began posturing itself and continued the development of an aggressive marketing plan to be put into action in the event the FDA would approve the use of Rezulin as a means to prevent diabetes.[17]

Margaret's Story

Pulling herself up from her knees, Margaret wiped tears that had spilled down her dark brown cheeks while praying. Her heart was heavy for those with chronic illnesses; she'd just been praying for them. She felt compelled to put her faith into action in some practical way within her community.

The next morning, Margaret looked up from the newspaper she'd been reading with her coffee. "Listen to this, Baby," she said to her husband without lifting her eyes from the page. She read to him about the Diabetes Prevention Program (DPP) sponsored by the local community hospital. The hospital was recruiting volunteers to participate in a study to see if taking a new drug, following a special diet, and keeping steady levels of exercise could actually decrease the risk of developing adult onset or Type II diabetes mellitus.[18]

After sharing life for thirty years, they didn't have need for words in moments like these. Clarence nodded. Many African Americans were struggling with diabetes in their neighborhood, and he knew his wife would help in any way she could, even if it meant volunteering to be a subject for research. He'd have to trust God on this one.

He was proud of his vibrant wife, who wore many hats serving those around her. How she managed everything, he'd never know. Not only was she the mother of his three kids, and a grandma too, she also taught history at the public school and Sunday school at their church, Zion Church of God. She took special interest in her students and was one of those teachers who knew how to encourage each student to do his or her best. She always nudged—well, maybe even pushed—her students, and they loved her for it.

Now that both of them were in their mid-fifties, Clarence marveled at his wife's strength of character as well as her level of energy. Margaret fit the requirements: she had preclinical diabetes shown by elevated fasting blood sugars. She didn't have actual diabetes yet and hadn't taken medication of any kind for many years, so she signed up as one of three thousand volunteers across the United States for the Diabetes Prevention Program.

News Flash: "U.S. government's top diabetes researcher helps guide a $150 million federal study involving the diabetes pill Rezulin while serving as a paid consultant for the drug's manufacturer, Warner-Lambert Co."

Dr. Richard Eastman, one of the top diabetes researchers who oversaw the NIH study, came under intense criticism when it was discovered that he was also on the payroll of Warner-Lambert. Dr. Eastman denied all charges of conflicting interest, and the study continued.[19]

No one but the program director knew whether the pills Margaret received were the real medication or a fake (a placebo). The first few weeks went by without any noticeable changes. Margaret kept up her typical pace and focused more on exercise. She felt great and figured she must have been chosen to take the placebo.

Clarence was not the least bit concerned when Margaret seemed to come down with a flu bug several weeks after she started taking the pills for the DPP research. But unlike the normal stomach flu, this didn't go away, and his wife got sicker. After the fourth day of persistent vomiting, Clarence grew alarmed. Monday he called to schedule an appointment with their personal physician.

By Tuesday, Margaret was so weak she could hardly walk into the doctor's exam room. After Dr. Williams finished the exam, he had his lab technician draw some blood and sent it to the lab. He advised Margaret to go home and rest after giving her a shot to reduce the vomiting, hoping that she would keep down some fluids.

Clarence received an urgent call from the doctor early the next morning, advising that Margaret be admitted to the hospital immediately due to the possibility of hepatitis. Dr. Williams asked if she'd been taking any prescription medication or over-the-counter drugs like Tylenol. Clarence put Margaret on the phone, and with a voice now raspy and thin, she informed the doctor that she was involved in the Diabetes Prevention Program through the hospital but did not have any idea what she was taking.

Dr. Williams called the program director of the DPP, stating that he needed to know exactly what the examiners had given Margaret.

"Your patient has been taking the new drug, Rezulin, Doctor," came the matter-of-fact reply.

The DPP director didn't exhibit any noticeable concern, but the doctor remembered seeing an article about the new drug in the *New England Journal of Medicine*. He searched through his library until he found the right issue. This is what he read: "Among the 2,510 patients who received Rezulin in combined North American clinical trials, 48 patients developed evidence of liver damage, as compared to 3 of 475 controlled patients who received a placebo."[20, 21]

Though almost all liver damage reversed once the drug was stopped, the editors of the medical journal recommended that the drug be discontinued in patients where liver enzymes were found to be increasing. "Although in most cases the liver enzymes returned to normal, a small group of patients could progress to severe liver damage."[22]

The physician knew if the viral hepatitis tests came back normal, chances were good that Margaret was reacting to the Rezulin pill. His suspicions were right. All the tests did come back normal, and Dr. Williams informed Margaret and her family that he believed she was reacting to the pill from the study. He was encouraged that the medical reports in the journal indicated she might slowly get better now that she had discontinued the medication.

Sadly, Margaret's determination to get well and pick up where she had left off wasn't enough. Her eyes and skin grew more yellow, and two days later a specialist informed the family that Margaret had gone into severe liver failure. They needed to consider placing her on the liver transplant list. Devastated, they agreed.

Dr. Williams spent nights researching and making connections so his patient would be first on the transplant list due to the seriousness of her situation. In spite of his determination to give his patient back her life, Margaret slipped in and out of a coma over the next few days.

A liver did become available, but Margaret never made it through surgery. The surgeons explained that her liver failure had also caused multiple organ failure, and there was nothing they could do to save her.

Since the NIH study was a nationwide clinical trial exploring the possibility of whether Rezulin could prevent diabetes, none of the patients in the trial even had diabetes. The NIH decided to pull Rezulin from the study because it had no way of protecting the other participants from the same fate as Margaret.

The Postmarketing Experience

On an October morning in 1997, Dr. Robert Misbin, an FDA diabetes specialist who had advocated the approval of Rezulin, received a disturbing phone call. A Warner-Lambert executive called to inform him of the first liver failures after Rezulin's release. "We knew the essential truth—that Rezulin could cause liver failure. There was potential for a disaster all along," said Misbin.[23]

Congress, pharmaceutical companies, and many special interest groups (AIDS and cancer patients) had pushed the FDA to approve all drugs more quickly, and now our nation would experience one of the most severe backlashes since the legislation. Rezulin became the nation's fastest-approved diabetes drug. The FDA was now left with the dilemma of how the agency would handle reports of deaths due to liver failure Rezulin caused.[24]

> There was potential for a disaster all along.

Together the officials at the FDA and Warner-Lambert devised a remedy within weeks of the first reported liver deaths—a simple change in the drug label. It read, "Rezulin patients should have their liver functions monitored by blood tests every two to three months during the first year of use."[25] The FDA and Warner-Lambert hoped blood testing for early signs of liver damage would alert patients early enough to stop the medication and avert organ failure.

The next blow to the new drug occurred when British officials withdrew Rezulin from the market on December 1, 1997. The British communicated their concerns to the American FDA, stating that the apparent incidence of serious toxicity was much greater than originally thought. The FDA countered this news by making another label change, recommending that physicians check liver tests every month for the first *six* months rather than every two to three months. A third label change followed shortly thereafter; it recommended liver testing every month for the first eight months.[26]

FDA officials focused on the possibility that the liver would heal itself once the drug was withdrawn. There was absolutely no clinical evidence, however, that even close monitoring of liver functions in patients who were taking Rezulin could protect them from permanent liver damage.[27]

The Heat Gets Hotter

In response to several investigative articles reported in the *Los Angeles Times*, the newly appointed FDA commissioner, Jane Henney, soon ordered a reevaluation of Rezulin. This assignment went to Dr. David Graham, the agency's leading expert in evaluating drugs already on the market. It didn't take long for Dr. Graham to compile an impressive list of statistics that incriminated Rezulin as deadly.

Dr. Graham's Research Findings on the New Drug Rezulin

- An estimated 430 or more Rezulin patients had suffered liver failure.
- Patients incurred 1,200 times more risk of liver failure by taking Rezulin.
- One of every 1,800 Rezulin patients could be expected to suffer liver failure, a far cry from the 1-in-100,000 risk claimed by Warner-Lambert.
- Regular liver monitoring offered no safety guarantee, primarily because Rezulin could so quickly and unpredictably damage the liver. This damage could even take place in a few days' time.
- In his follow-up studies, Dr. Graham found that 99 percent of the patients who had been taking Rezulin for periods of greater than four months failed to follow the FDA liver-monitoring recommendations. [28]

As you might expect, Warner-Lambert's representatives assured the advisory committee that, contrary to Graham's findings, Rezulin was not responsible for many of the liver failures. They cited several factors, but the most persuasive argument was the fact that many of these patients had preexisting medical conditions.

The FDA advisory committee chose to ignore Dr. Graham's warnings and voted eleven to one to keep Rezulin on the market. Interestingly, three of the committee members were receiving compensation from

Warner-Lambert or an affiliate. How was that possible? They were granted conflict-of-interest waivers by the FDA![29]

It didn't take long before more deaths were reported due to liver failure in patients taking Rezulin. The FDA agreed to yet another labeling change, which would be the fourth since its release. Instead of renouncing the drug once and for all to prevent any further dangerous side effects, the FDA approved use of Rezulin in more clinical situations. By doing so, the FDA actually promoted the use of the diabetes drug rather than discouraging it.

Dr. Graham continued to compile strong arguments for the immediate withdrawal of Rezulin from the market. The agency had by this time confirmed eighty-five cases of liver failure, which included fifty-eight deaths.[30]

How Do You Stop This Train?

After the drug's release, its marketing momentum only heightened. Promises had been made, economic powers were hanging in the balance, and careers were on the line. This time Dr. Misbin (an FDA diabetes specialist who formerly advocated the approval of Rezulin) put himself at risk. The FDA could no longer dance around the danger of Rezulin.

Going *outside* the agency with sensitive interagency e-mails and reports, Misbin put himself in harm's way with the agency. Dr. Misbin wrote to Rep. Henry A. Waxman (D-Los Angeles) and seven other lawmakers. He knew his actions would put constraint on the top executives at the FDA. More meetings were soon held, and Dr. Graham had another chance to share his concerns with the top officials in the agency. Conclusive evidence was in—the longer patients remained on Rezulin, the greater their risk of developing liver toxicity.[31]

The FDA finally announced Warner-Lambert's voluntary withdrawal of Rezulin from the market on March 21, 2000—nearly thirty months after the first reported case of liver failure in a patient taking Rezulin, and twenty-eight months after Britain pulled Rezulin from its market. Upon the FDA's request, Warner-Lambert voluntarily withdrew Rezulin from the market, stating there were safer alternatives now on the market. [32]

What Does All This Mean?

The Rezulin story provides documented evidence of a drug's history. From preclinical trials through fast-track approval process, marketing blitzes, postmarket surveillance, and finally withdrawal, you can trace the influences of the powers that be. When a drug runs into problems, and hundreds or even thousands of people are innocently injured or killed, there is certainly enough blame to go around. Undoubtedly, following the withdrawal of Rezulin, it's easy to point to the underlying problems of an accelerated drug-approval process spurred on by massive marketing strategies and the economic stakes in postmarketing surveillance.

Rezulin was a brand-new, novel approach to the treatment of Type II diabetes. Millions of patients hoped to use this drug for a lifetime and even prevent diabetes altogether. Warner-Lambert appeared to have a winner in every aspect of its new drug.

In the short time Rezulin was on the market, it generated $2.1 billion in sales.[33] Warner-Lambert presented everything the FDA required. This means presenting data, clinical trials, animal-testing results, and effectiveness of its drug. The FDA merely reviews the data presented to it.

Many times the FDA will approve a drug for the market while placing a nonbinding requirement for postmarket studies. In the case of Rezulin, Warner-Lambert was to do a clinical trial in patients with heart problems to be sure that Rezulin did not cause further heart damage. However, this study was never completed.

Over the years, as a physician, I have seen a pattern when it comes to statements made by pharmaceutical companies regarding reports to the FDA about potential serious problems with their drugs. Since the FDA has a voluntary reporting system, companies will first state that it was not the drug that actually caused complications but rather an underlying disease process that the patient already had. Since there is no way to really prove them wrong, this response usually suppresses critics.

When reports of death or serious adverse drug reactions continue and there is no way to further deny that its drug is the problem, a company's most common response is to state that it is a very rare occur-

It is important for you never to forget that there are risks for every drug.

rence. In the case of Rezulin, the company commented several times that it felt the incidence of liver failure occurred in fewer than 1 in 100,000 cases. Who could prove it wrong?

It is important for you never to forget that there are risks for every drug. The FDA certainly never does! In fact, it never expects everyone on the drug advisory committee to agree on the drug's safety. There are always problems or potential problems with every drug. If the agency needed a unanimous decision to get every drug approved, none ever would be.

The voluntary reporting system for adverse drug reactions offers the FDA plenty of breathing room to protect its original decision to approve a drug. Again, since there is no way to truly know how frequently a serious drug reaction is occurring, the FDA simply needs to make changes in the labeling information on the drug. This is what happened in the case of Rezulin—four different times. This is the FDA's greatest defense when adverse effects get serious, as was the case with Rezulin.

Dr. Janet Woodcock was quoted in the *Los Angeles Times* as saying, "The agency's [FDA] objective in keeping Rezulin on the market for 29 months following the first reported liver failure deaths was to empower doctors to make their own, informed judgments. It wasn't that people [doctors] were compelled to prescribe this drug. People could also choose not to take the drug. Doctors and patients have to make choices. And we at the FDA want them to be as informed as possible." [34]

The Rezulin story is a disturbing one. For you the reader, there are some basic truths you must take away from this devastating chain of events: All drugs are inherently dangerous. Putting blind faith in the system that has gone wrong could cost you or your loved ones a life. This is only one example of a drug that the FDA quickly approved and then withdrew within a few years.

Unfortunately, Rezulin is not the only tragic drug story. In fact, millions of patients in the United States alone took at least one of the five drugs withdrawn from the market between September 1997 and September 1998.

The FDA claims the drug-approval system is working. Are you convinced? In upcoming chapters I will present additional stories of individual drugs withdrawn from the market.

CHAPTER SIX

A System Gone Wrong

AT ITS BEST, OUR DRUG-APPROVAL SYSTEM IS FAR FROM FAIL-safe. Not only does it heavily involve you, the general public, to test new drugs; but also with the driving urgency of having medications approved on shorter time lines, dangerous loopholes have developed. We know the margin of error has broadened as a result of the FDA's releasing an onslaught of new drugs. We realize our dependence on a voluntary reporting system where only limited FDA staff and funds monitor postmarketing drug surveillance. Still, physicians continue practicing medicine as they always have—acting in good faith, hoping everything will turn out all right.

The office of Postmarketing Drug Risk Assessment has an overwhelming task before it. Compared to the more than 1,400 employees with the principal duties of approving new drugs, the FDA staffs only 65 full-time employees who are responsible for monitoring the 8,000 brand-name, generic, and over-the-counter drugs already on the market today. This department includes fewer than 10 individuals with either a Ph.D. or M.D. degree.[1]

The odds are not in our favor. The new legislation in 1997 introduced several standards of drug approval and use that brought flexibility, easier access . . . and the off-label use of drugs. As a result of not adequately acknowledging the heavy consequences of our recent legislation, doctors are contributing players in a system gone wrong.

Baby Sarah's Story

At age twenty-four Katie married her childhood sweetheart, and together they developed a successful brokerage business. While still in college, she and Beau had dreamed about their first home and the family they would someday share. Dreams did come true, and the newlyweds closed on their first little starter house in Elk Grove, a new housing division just outside of town.

Like many young couples, Katie and her husband wanted to postpone having children until their financial situation became reliable. After being married three years, Beau and Katie's careers were stable, and they felt settled in. The garage (instead of the second bedroom) now stored their bikes, kayaks, and camping gear. They finished putting in the landscaping and privacy fence. They were ready.

Katie was ecstatic when she became pregnant in the second month of trying. She counted her blessings, hoping against any problems during the pregnancy. Katie chose the décor and Beau fixed up the nursery in periwinkle blue and yellow. The final touch was hanging a smiling moon over the crib. As the due date drew near, Katie stacked tiny diapers and sleepers in the new changing table. She couldn't wait to inhale the soft baby smell of her newborn. She and Beau took Lamaze classes, making a commitment to having their baby naturally— without the use of *any* drugs.

The day arrived four weeks earlier than they had planned, and the labor was tough and long. Katie's doctor was great, though, and Beau was a trooper. The baby was born after twenty hours of labor, arriving with a loud cry and alert eyes. True to her plan, Katie made it through her entire labor without any medication. How thrilled she and Beau were to hear the words they had waited for so long: "Mr. and Mrs. Zohne, you now have a beautiful, healthy girl."

Even though she was early, baby Sarah went home with her new proud parents after twenty-four hours. Katie decided to breast-feed, because she knew this was the best thing for her little one. She took a six-month leave from work and even had thoughts of quitting work entirely to stay home with Sarah. Being a mother was more wonderful than she could have ever imagined possible. While rocking the baby and stroking her silky hair, Katie dreamed of the joys she and Beau would share as their daughter grew.

By the time little Sarah had reached two months old, she was socializing and smiling. She seemed to learn something new every day. At her two-month well-baby checkup the pediatrician announced that she was perfectly healthy. The baby's only problem was the tendency to spit up a lot after her feedings. The pediatrician said he was not at all concerned. The baby was gaining weight, and the spitting up, though a nuisance, was definitely nothing serious and would most likely stop before Sarah turned one year of age. He advised Katie to burp her more frequently and not worry.

By three months of age, however, Sarah was spitting up after each feeding in spite of frequent burping, and she had stopped gaining weight, which concerned Katie and Beau. They again visited the pediatrician, who reassured them that this condition was a minor problem of reflux seen frequently in babies. The doctor then suggested they try giving Sarah a new drug, Propulsid, as part of a study; it was effective in controlling acid reflux in young children. He listed the potential minor symptoms that could arise, but he explained the drug was safe for use in infants and would control Sarah's problem until she reached twelve months.

Though the young parents were not prone to use any drugs, their hopes rose at the possibility of being involved in a study that could help their baby. They were tired of mopping up sour spit-up and felt embarrassed when others didn't want to hold Sarah for fear she would make a mess. Beau and Katie agreed to participate. They distinctly remember being comforted by the consent form stating that the FDA had approved Propulsid for use in children.

After Beau and Katie went through the formality of answering some questions and receiving precautions about the use of the new drug, their pediatrician informed them that the risks were minimal and handed them a bottle with the medication already prepared. You can imagine their relief when Sarah quit spitting up after her feedings. She seemed to tolerate the medication well and continued to grow and develop normally.

On a warm fall evening in late October, Beau and Katie kissed Sarah's chubby baby cheeks as they put her to bed on her four-month birthday. Pulling the string to start a little music box playing at the side of her crib, they whispered, "Good night, little darling."

Off-Label Use of Propulsid

As in the case of Sarah's pediatrician, all doctors find themselves in the difficult position of having to decide whether a drug is safe for their patients. Pediatricians, however, have had to use adult medications for years without the benefit of conclusive clinical trials. Because drug investigators do not typically conduct trials on children, doctors are left to guess the proper prescription doses for infant patients.

As you will recall, congress passed the FDAMA (1997) legislation in part to help correct this problem, therefore encouraging pharmaceutical companies to conduct clinical trials with children. If drug companies agreed to perform these trials, the FDA would in turn extend the company's patent an additional six months. Unfortunately, Propulsid's manufacturer did not take this option.

Nevertheless, Propulsid was widely used for infants. Many pediatricians prescribed the drug to treat babies like Sarah with gastroesophageal reflux to stop them from spitting up or vomiting after their feedings. You see, we don't actually have a valve to hold food in the stomach. Babies, as well as adults, rely on what is called lower esophageal pressure, which usually prevents this reflux of acid. However, in premature newborn infants, this lower esophageal pressure is poorly developed, and it is very common to have reflux.

Infants with this reflux problem may actually lose weight or struggle to gain properly. Though the FDA had never approved Propulsid for use in children, and this was thus considered an off-label use, the drug was very effective in correcting the reflux condition and its use spread rapidly among pediatricians. One follow-up survey showed that of fifty-eight thousand premature babies, 20 percent received Propulsid.[2]

Postmarketing Surveillance Falls Short

Are you familiar with the medical term, *QT interval*? The QT interval is the period of time it takes for one's heart ventricles (the large pumping muscles) to contract and relax, usually taking about four-tenths of a second. If this time interval is extended even slightly, it can cause a disruption of the normal heart rhythm and may even lead to a sudden cardiac arrest.

Some people are born with a slightly prolonged QT interval, meaning they are at a greater risk for cardiac rhythm problems—especially when taking certain drugs. Several medications currently on the market (including some antibiotics) are known to prolong the QT interval. When a patient is taking two or more of these drugs, or when the patient's QT interval is already prolonged, the results may prove lethal.

QT Interval

Dr. Andre Dubois, an FDA medical officer who reviewed a premarket clinical trial involving nearly 2,000 patients, discovered that 48 of the patients experienced heart rhythm problems as a direct result of Propulsid prolonging the QT interval.[3]

It is important to understand how the drug Propulsid affected the QT interval. First, let's go back to the drug's origins. In 1993, when the FDA considered approval of the heartburn medication Propulsid, it knew that the drug could accentuate this QT interval problem and possibly lead to a patient's death. Though FDA officials were aware of the life-threatening risk, they approved the new medication in July of that same year with a warning *on the 135th line of fine print in the drug's label.*[4]

> Though FDA officials were aware of the life-threatening risk, they approved the new medication with a warning on the 135th line of fine print in the drug's label.

Shortly after the release of Propulsid, the FDA began receiving reports of patients experiencing heart irregularities and even death due to cardiac arrest after taking the new drug. Still, the pharmaceutical company strongly denied that any of these deaths were a direct cause of the new medication. Responding predictably, the FDA endorsed the first of *five* labeling changes to the product information packet.[5]

———

Katie rolled over with aching breasts full of milk. She squinted with sleepy eyes at the clock. It read 6:30 A.M. With a sense of dread, she knew something was wrong; she'd missed the night feeding because Sarah had not cried or fussed all night. Panicked, Katie stumbled to the baby's room and flipped on the light. Grabbing the infant, she found her cold and stiff. *"No!* No, no, no, no!" she screamed. Beau came running.

Baby Sarah was dead.

Unaware of the medication she'd been given, the coroner listed Sarah's cause of death as SIDS, or Sudden Infant Death Syndrome. Like Beau and Katie, many people at first believed their infants' deaths were a result of SIDS because Propulsid deaths mimicked the well-known killer of infants. This is what makes discovering adverse drug reactions so difficult—they may resemble similar common diseases or problems.

Beau and Katie's grief seemed unbearable. Once a room filled with hope and new life, the nursery now cradled only emptiness and grief. Days blurred together, and weeks passed. Three months after Sarah's death, Beau read an article in the local newspaper announcing the removal of Propulsid from the market due to a large number of reported deaths in adults and children. Feeling sick in the pit of his stomach, he knew the truth. Researching everything he could find on the drug, he soon discovered that many children had died of cardiac arrest while taking the drug.[6] Much to his dismay, he also learned that *the FDA had never actually approved Propulsid for use in children*. Physicians were simply using it off-label in children.

Feverishly Beau dug through the medical file at home until he found a copy of the consent form he and Katie had signed at the doc-

> How tragic and unnecessary were these deaths.

tor's office. He could see nothing in the label warnings about the potential risk of cardiac arrest. The only adverse side effects listed were minor problems such as diarrhea, bloating, or possible abdominal pain. The document failed to mention that this drug was being used apart from what the FDA approved it for—or that death could result.

Beau immediately contacted the pediatrician and asked to see him personally. The doctor was quick to respond to the grieving father's concerns about the drug he had prescribed for baby Sarah; but he was adamant that he had verbally warned the young parents of the possibility of death with the use of the drug even though the consent form did not spell it out. When asked why the consent form indicated that the FDA had approved Propulsid for use in children, the physician simply shrugged, saying it had obviously been an oversight.

Finally—Propulsid Was Removed from the Market

In August of 1996, after receiving reports of twenty children who had suffered heart rhythm disturbances in addition to reports of eleven deaths due to cardiac arrest, the FDA contacted the maker of Propulsid to specifically inform it the drug *was no longer approved* for off-label use in children. Unfortunately, due to a breakdown in the system, neither physicians nor patients learned of the FDA's concerns regarding the use of the drug in children.[7] In fact, a revised label change acknowledging several pediatric deaths was not formally made until June 1998, twenty-two months later.

Like Beau and Katie, parents of children who died during this time exclaimed during interviews that they had no idea the drug could potentially cause cardiac arrest. If parents had been informed of the potential risk of sudden death when their child used this drug, I am sure many of them would never have consented to their infant's use of Propulsid. How tragic and unnecessary were these deaths, especially when reflux corrects itself 95 percent of the time before a child reaches the age of one year.

At the time the FDA forced the manufacturer to remove Propulsid from the market in July of 2000, voluntary reports had cited it as suspect in more than three hundred deaths since its approval seven years prior. Many deaths involved infants.[8] Dr. Florence Houn, an official with the FDA, was quoted as saying, "We've had a seven year history with this drug and it has been *a rich opportunity for us to learn*. One of the things we have learned is the approved indication for a drug really needs to justify the serious and life-threatening side effects" (italics mine).[9] In effect, Houn stated that using a drug for heartburn when it can potentially cause sudden death doesn't make much sense.

Many dynamics are at work here. First, there is always the inherent risk of all medications. Second, in the case of Propulsid, could the FDA have acted more quickly and more effectively in warning physicians or withdrawing Propulsid from the market? Pediatricians are frequently under the gun to find safe and effective medications for their young patients, making the use of adult drugs off-label a common and necessary practice. This demands nothing less than clear and open communication between the FDA and the physician. Consequently, the Food and Drug Administration was not the only one that possibly needed to share the blame. The third dynamic contributing to a system gone wrong was a failure at the level of the doctor's office.

The third dynamic contributing to a system gone wrong was a failure at the level of the doctor's office.

Sharing the Blame

You know the old saying, "It takes two to tango." Communication is always a two-way street, and warnings cannot be effective if no one heeds them. In the case of Propulsid, Janet Woodcock, the FDA's director of drug evaluation, admitted the FDA's fault in not formally weighing the risk of the drug's off-label use while keeping it on the market.[10]

Acknowledging that it was indeed prescribed widely for children, she *still* held physicians responsible for making prudent decisions. "Once a drug is proved safe and effective," said Woodcock, "the FDA depends on doctors to take into account the risks, to read the label. . . . We have to rely on the practitioner community to be the learned intermediary. That is why drugs are prescription drugs."[11]

When trouble comes one's way, it's easy to pass the buck so that the next link in the chain receives the blame—and this time fingers pointed at physicians. I must admit that Woodcock made an important point. The public does rely on practitioners to read labels and mediate on behalf of their patients. How well *are* doctors doing their jobs in regard to knowing prescription medications?

In the December 20, 2000 issue of the *Journal of the American Medical Association,* a study addressed whether doctors properly heeded warnings from the FDA in regard to the dangers of Propulsid. This study indicated what I already knew to be true—most physicians are not reading package inserts or paying close attention to the FDA warnings on "Dear Health-Care Professional" letters.[12]

After the FDA released Propulsid in 1993, its manufacturer aggressively marketed it to physicians. And in 1995, doctors wrote approximately five *million* prescriptions for Propulsid in the United States alone. By 1995 more than thirty reported cases of heart-rhythm problems and four deaths had been reported. In response, the FDA added a "black box" to the drug's label, warning physicians not to give patients the drug if they were taking other medications that would affect its metabolism. (The main concern here was that many drugs were metabolized—see Chapter 8—the same way as Propulsid. Therefore, when a patient took these types of drugs at the same time he was receiving Propulsid, it would increase the blood levels of Propulsid and, therefore, increase the risk of sudden death.) The pharmaceutical company also issued a "Dear Health-Care Professional" letter to warn physicians of this potential hazard. [13]

Despite the "black box" warning, use of Propulsid grew, and in 1998 pharmacies dispensed more than seven million scripts for the drug. Clinical studies at that time showed conclusive evidence that the new drug did in fact prolong the QT interval of healthy volunteers. During the time period the FDA was receiving this research information, it was also receiving more and more reports of deaths from Propulsid. The FDA again added additional warnings to the label as well as distributing yet another "Dear Doctor" letter. In fact, the FDA sent out eight hundred thousand letters to physicians, pharmacists, and vendors of drug-alert databases. [14]

The *JAMA* study concluded that in the twelve months following the FDA's intensive regulatory action, more than 40 percent of all new Propulsid prescriptions were written for patients for whom the FDA did not recommend the drug, which placed them directly "in harm's way." [15]

The exposure of these patients to inappropriate use of Propulsid, *despite the prominent publication* of case reports, label changes, and "Dear Health-Care Professional" letters, demonstrates the total ineffectiveness of FDA warnings in a system gone wrong. Needless to say, physicians were not paying attention or responding to FDA warnings. Propulsid was finally removed from the market in July 2000.

> The exposure of these patients to inappropriate use of Propulsid demonstrates the total ineffectiveness of FDA warnings in a system gone wrong.

Don't Have Blind Faith in Your Physician

Propulsid was a drug for heartburn. It was not created for a life-or-death situation. In spite of the fact that several other safer alternatives were available, doctors prescribed it—and hundreds of deaths were reported to the FDA during the seven years and five label changes this drug was on the market. FDA officials attempted to notify physicians with warnings about possible serious adverse reactions, but as we've seen, the findings of the *JAMA* study prove that few paid attention.

In spite of the fact that several other safer alternatives were available, hundreds of deaths were reported to the FDA during the seven years and five label changes this drug was on the market.

As you have seen in the case of Propulsid and Rezulin, and as you will see later in the case of Duract, physicians are *not* paying adequate attention to warnings and label changes the FDA releases. I like to ask pharmaceutical representatives who visit my office if they believe physicians actually read in their entirety the numerous package-insert labels they leave for us. Their response is universally the same—they just laugh and say something like, "Are you kidding me?" When I ask how many doctors they feel actually read the drug label completely, the response is almost always the same: "None, or maybe 1 percent." In America, the medical community as well as its patients must wake up to the reality that we've entered a whole new era of medicine. Our passivity is no longer good enough.

I find the reality of participating in a "trial" we know nothing about deeply troubling, especially when it involves a little child like Sarah. Even more disturbing is the knowledge that patients can possibly find themselves in dangerous predicaments when doctors do not heed warnings—they are the professionals in whom patients place their trust. How shall we live when "black box" warnings and "Dear Doctor" letters fall by the wayside in the busy worlds of most physicians—when the system fails to work?

Aggressive communication is key. And the responsibility is yours as well as your doctor's. You cannot rely solely on your doctor to tell you all the potential problems that may occur with the medication he or she is about to prescribe. Instead, you must become informed about the potential problems your medication may cause and, even then, listen very carefully to your body. When you feel something is not right, pay close attention, and at least consider the possibilty of a drug reaction—

known or unknown. Second, you must be bold enough to discuss your concerns with your physician whenever you feel that you may be reacting to any medication. I will cover in detail in Chapter 13 how to best protect yourself from an adverse drug reaction.

If your doctor is unwilling to discuss your options, you should consider finding one who is. In contrast to the tragic outcome of baby Sarah's story, the following is an example of how a patient took an active role in saving himself from a life-threatening adverse drug reaction.

Bill's Story

Bill worked hard to support his family in his career as a gourmet chef in metropolitan Denver. He and his wife, Mary, believed it was important that she stay home with the children, so they arranged their budget to live totally on Bill's income. Bill took time to exercise regularly. He also ate well and enjoyed preparing meals for his family when time allowed.

During one of the busier days at the restaurant, Bill needed to lift a heavy sack of rice from the floor onto the table. As he lifted the bag, he immediately felt a pain in his back so severe it brought him to his knees. That night Bill couldn't sleep, even after taking acetaminophen.

> You cannot rely solely on your doctor to tell you all the potential problems with the medication he or she is about to prescribe.

Hardly able to move, Bill went to see his doctor the next morning. When the doctor found no evidence of a herniated disc, he concluded that Bill had most likely strained his back. This was not the first time his patient had been in as a result of back pain. Once or twice a year Bill injured his back, and it seemed to grow weaker with each occurrence.

The family doctor instructed Bill to start on muscle relaxants. He suggested that Bill try a new pain medication that had just been released a few months earlier. In fact, he told Bill he had personally tried Duract for his own back strain from a golfing injury. The doctor said that it worked great and was safe because it was a nonsteroidal, anti-inflammatory medication like Motrin and Aleve. Unlike others, Duract was much more effective in its ability to relieve pain.

He wrote the script for Duract and gave Bill several refills in case he needed to take the medication for a while. Bill went home and began taking the Duract along with the muscle relaxant. He slowly improved over the next few days and was finally able to go back to work a week later. His back was still hurting, but he found that if he took the Duract, he didn't feel groggy and he didn't have much pain. As soon as the Duract would wear off, however, the pain would start to intensify.

About three weeks later, Bill developed what he thought was the flu. He became sick to his stomach and even vomited a couple times one day. His appetite disappeared, and he began to lose some weight. Each day he thought he might feel better, but after about a month he was down fifteen pounds. He became concerned that the nausea was so persistent. He realized that something was definitely wrong—this was not a case of the flu.

Carefully reading the information the pharmacist had given him on the new drug Duract, he found a startling warning: *the medication should be used only for acute pain and not for any period longer than five to ten days.*

This information came as a shock to Bill. His doctor had specifically given him instructions to continue taking the medication as needed and had even provided several refills! He also noticed that the insert mentioned abdominal discomfort, nausea, and even jaundice as warning signs of a reaction to the medication. After Bill read this he immediately quit taking the Duract and made an appointment to see his doctor.

At his appointment, Bill described the nausea and weight loss. His doctor showed concern and decided to run some blood tests as well as an upper GI series to be sure his patient hadn't developed an ulcer from the Duract. When the results came back from the tests, he set an appointment with Bill and Mary for a consultation. Fearing they might receive news of cancer, they were deeply concerned.

The doctor showed Bill the results of the tests and x-rays. Surprisingly, his stomach was perfectly normal. The bad news was still to come. Next, they discussed Bill's chemistry profile, which showed high elevation of his liver enzymes. The doctor was not sure what was causing his patient's liver problems, but he was definitely alarmed that the readings were so high. He suggested that Bill see a gastroenterologist for further tests and a possible liver biopsy. Bill couldn't believe what he was hearing. He didn't drink alcohol and rarely took medication except for the times when his back would go out.

Bill figured now was the time to mention the precautions he'd read about the Duract. At first, the doctor said that he didn't think this was the problem. But Bill persisted. He'd brought the Duract information with him. After reading the warnings for the use of the new drug, the physician blanched. He admitted his patient directly into the hospital.

After Bill's complete evaluation by the local GI specialist, he learned that he had severe liver failure, most likely caused by the Duract. The risk of liver damage did, in fact, significantly increase when a patient took the drug for periods longer than ten days.[16] Bill was in trouble.

He had a difficult next two weeks, but his liver enzymes finally began to improve. He started to get his appetite back and was even beginning to gain a little weight. Fortunately, he fully recovered, and in the end he had no residual complications.

In retrospect, Bill distinctly remembers the remark his gastroenterologist made as he was being discharged from the hospital. Shaking his head, the specialist said, "Bill, if you had not been suspicious of the medication as the cause of your symptoms and had not stopped taking Duract when you did, I don't believe you would have survived."

Bill's doctor was not alone in overlooking the warnings for Duract. The FDA was forced to ask the makers of Duract to remove the drug from the market because hundreds of doctors were not heeding its warnings of its short-term use. In fact, doctors would frequently write prescriptions for Duract with several refills. And the FDA received sixty-eight voluntary reports of suspected deaths due to Duract. [17]

Best Voluntary Reporting in the World?

Bill's adverse drug event resulted from a physician's error—not using the drug properly according to the FDA's warnings in prescribing a short-term prescription medication with refills over too long a period. With rigorously scheduled days and a focus primarily on disease rather than adverse drug reactions, most doctors are apparently too busy to read all the warning labels. How then can we anticipate that physicians will readily recognize and report an adverse drug reaction when it occurs? Still the FDA considers our reporting system the "best" voluntary system in the world. [18]

One might think that hospital staffs, with all of their personnel and the frequency with which they see serious adverse drug reactions, would be the best source from which to gather information or the most keen-eyed observers when it comes to ADRs. On the contrary; hospitals have strong incentives not to identify too many of these events. After all, reporting large numbers of drug reactions or events brings intense scrutiny from both regulators and the public.

Hospital staff members, who also rely on spontaneous voluntary reporting, report only approximately one in twenty adverse drug reactions.[19] This ultimately leads to the perception by physicians and the public that prescription-drug-induced injuries are less common than they really are.

The lack of reporting may also be due to the limited training of medical students in clinical pharmacology and therapeutics. Doctors simply do not receive sufficient training in pharmacology or the use of medication. Of the 120 medical schools surveyed, 100 of them only offered a one-semester course in pharmacology, and that was early in the medical students' training. In short, medical schools do not encourage physicians to become adequately trained in recognizing possible drug reactions.[20] When all of these factors are combined, you see why there is such serious delay in discovering adverse drug reactions of newly released drugs.

MedWatch

Since 1993, the FDA has attempted to make reporting of adverse drug events easier through the MedWatch Program. This new system encourages health-care professionals to regard reporting as a fundamental professional and public health responsibility. It sounds nice. But it has done little to improve the number of reports the FDA receives.[21]

An article in *JAMA* (1998) reported that in spite of the MedWatch program, still only 1 percent of all serious adverse drug reactions are ever reported to the FDA by doctors. (The FDA received only 3,863 [5.2 percent] of 73,887 reports directly from physicians in 1994.) Furthermore, spontaneous reporting of drug reactions proves difficult or even impossible in trying to estimate *how often* a particular reaction actually occurs.[22]

One of my close physician friends shared with me how he reported what he believed was a serious drug reaction. The FDA rewarded him for his straightforward concern with an overwhelming load of paperwork and frequent contact. After wading through piles of pages to report an ADR to the pharmaceutical rep, he became so frustrated that he clearly stated he was never going to report another. Unfortunately, this is the usual attitude physicians have toward reporting known reactions, even with the helpful changes made in the MedWatch Program, such as providing a simple, one-page report to use when reporting suspected adverse reactions.

Stories like baby Sarah's are deeply troubling because many of us have parents, friends, or a spouse who has been touched by a frightening drug reaction and perhaps even a tragedy. Has our system gone wrong? Undoubtedly. Are we destined to become its victims? Absolutely not. Bill's story demonstrates otherwise. He took a chance in discontinuing his medication and pursued help right away—even when he had to confront his doctor and challenge him to read the warnings he had in hand. I believe you can be confident in and proactive about protecting yourself from an adverse drug reaction as well. I'll tell you how in the pages to come.

CHAPTER SEVEN

Clear and Present Danger

I'VE SPOKEN OF THE REALITY THAT EVERY DRUG COMES WITH both benefits and risks. But you must know: benefit versus risk is a relative concept. It is true, every drug has some risk and every drug the FDA approves has some potential benefit; however, *all drugs are inherently dangerous*.

The severity of the disease that a drug has been developed to treat will determine exactly how much risk the FDA may be willing for you to accept. For example, if you suffer from degenerative arthritis and receive a drug that caused all of your hair to fall out, you will not be a happy camper. But on the other hand, if you are dying of cancer and take a chemotherapeutic drug that causes all of your hair to fall out—and extends your life—you will most likely accept the risk.

Every drug that the FDA considers for approval must offer a significantly greater benefit than risk, but undeniable risk always remains. As I've said, every time a physician prescribes a medication, he must weigh the benefit of a particular drug against the risk that drug may cause to the patient. But they, as well as trusting patients, place far too much faith in the benefits of drugs and don't take enough caution in regard to their potential danger.

Bob's Story

At sixty-one years of age, Bob has coronary artery disease and will never walk again. His heart problems have little to do with his muscle weakness, but medication sure does.

Two years ago Bob suffered a major heart attack that required open-heart surgery for a double bypass procedure. He seemed to bounce back well, and the doctor was optimistic about her patient's future. The only drawback was that Bob's cholesterol was still elevated. His total cholesterol was 265, and his LDL, or "bad" cholesterol, was 178—it should have been below 100. The cardiologist informed Bob that he needed to work *aggressively* at lowering his cholesterol. She was confident that diet alone would not do the trick and recommended that Bob take a "statin" drug, which is a potent cholesterol-lowering drug.

The cardiologist started Bob on a statin drug called Baycol with a 0.4 mg dosage at bedtime. She mentioned no precautions about the use of the drug. All she said was that Bob should get another chemistry profile, which checks for diabetes, liver function, kidney function, and cholesterol, in eight weeks to see how his body was responding to the medication.

All drugs are inherently dangerous.

Bob slowly regained his strength after the surgery and was able to return to work three months later, feeling great. Several good months passed, and it was again time to visit the cardiologist for his six-month checkup. The heart patient walked with a brisk step. Because he'd been eating carefully and exercising consistently, he was actually in better shape than before the heart attack.

Bob's total cholesterol had improved somewhat, dropping to 210, but his LDL cholesterol had dropped only to 134. With a concerned look, the cardiologist went to her free-sample cabinet, brought back a newly released 0.8 mg dose of Baycol, and handed it to Bob.

Without a second thought, Bob started taking the higher dose of Baycol that night. During the months of recovery following his heart attack, he would lay awake, pondering how the doctors and medical staff had come together so perfectly with all their knowledge and skills to orchestrate a new chance for life. He was filled with gratitude and never thought for a minute of questioning the cardiologist's judgment on something as routine as a prescription.

Initially Bob didn't notice any changes and continued to feel well; but after a few weeks, he began experiencing stabbing pains in both hips. In just a few days, he grew worried about the growing weakness in both legs and then in both arms. His cardiologist could not figure out what was happening and admitted Bob to the hospital. She consulted a neurologist, anticipating that Bob had suffered a stroke.

The neurologist conducted a battery of tests during the first two days of his hospitalization and soon discovered that Bob was reacting to his statin medication, Baycol. The recovering heart patient had developed a rare complication called rhabdomyolysis (a serious breakdown and destruction of muscle). The Baycol had caused his muscle cells to die, and the waste products from the muscle were being spewed into his bloodstream. Though his kidneys were trying to clear these toxic wastes from the bloodstream, Bob went into kidney failure within the next twenty-four hours. Renal dialysis was the only option after his body started shutting down.

Bob's wife, Sandy, could not believe how horrible he looked. In just a few days his skin became dry and wrinkled, and his muscles looked like they had shrunk away. Her husband was unable to move any part of his body except his fingers and toes. His potassium had risen to such dangerously high levels, the internist who took over his case informed Sandy that Bob was not likely to live but a day or two longer.

After Sandy heard this devastating prognosis from Bob's physician, she called several key people who had been praying for Bob from the time he had become ill. Their only hope now was divine intervention by the Great Healer. The medical staff was baffled when Bob started feeling better, and over the next couple of days his kidney function began improving for the first time. A week later he was sitting up and eating by himself. Three weeks later, still unable to walk, he was discharged to go home.

Bob spent many months recovering from his harrowing near-death experience with the cholesterol-lowering drug Baycol. You can imagine his response when three months following his discharge from the hospital, Baycol's manufacturer took it off the market. The FDA issued a statement that the drug had been incriminated in thirty-one deaths due to rhabdomyolysis.[1] Bob shuddered, knowing he had almost been number thirty-two.

Gratitude for being alive then turned to righteous anger. Yes, God has spared Bob's life, but his cardiologist had never once mentioned that rhabdomyolysis could be a potential problem. In fact, when Bob first consulted the specialist about his muscle weakness, she didn't know what was taking place. "I would go through ten heart attacks before I would ever go through something like this again!" exclaimed Bob. "That drug should never have been approved."

Statin Drugs

Do you have high cholesterol? Pharmaceutical companies are betting that you do. Twelve million patients are presently taking statin drugs for elevated cholesterol. Yet such companies claim that only one-third of the population that needs to be on these drugs is actually taking them.[2] Their reps are continually encouraging doctors to get more patients on statin drugs.

In fact, pharmaceutical companies are delighted that the government has lowered the recommended safe level of LDL cholesterol to 100, which previously was 130. Almost 90 percent of my patients now have *apparent* elevated cholesterol levels because of what I believe are unrealistic recommended levels of LDL cholesterol. Physicians are now placing their patients on statin drugs at unprecedented frequency.

> Almost 90 percent of my patients now have *apparent* elevated cholesterol levels because of what I believe are unrealistic recommended levels of LDL cholesterol.

Before you call your doctor to schedule a checkup on your cholesterol levels, you should know that health-care professionals still believe that every patient deserves a trial of diet and exercise prior to starting any cholesterol-lowering drug. Still, *most* physicians find it easier to merely give lip service to this recommendation while writing out prescriptions for statin drugs.

In my most recent book, *What Your Doctor Doesn't Know About Nutritional Medicine May Be Killing You* (Thomas Nelson Publishers, 2002), I explain in detail how heart disease is an inflammatory disease of the artery and *not* a disease of cholesterol. Contrary to popular belief, researchers have found that more than half of the patients who have heart attacks in this country have normal cholesterol levels. Furthermore, they have discovered that not all cholesterol is detrimental to our health. Only the "oxidized" or "modified" LDL cholesterol is bad—not our native or natural LDL cholesterol.

(Note: Cellular nutrition is critical in decreasing or eliminating all the causes of inflammation of the artery. If you have elevated cholesterol levels, I strongly encourage you to read this book to gain a fuller understanding of how you can best protect your arteries.)

A History of Baycol

Bob illustrated the dangers behind what the FDA called the promising new "lifesaving drug." Premarketing trials had tested it on more than three thousand patients, and the FDA approved Baycol in 1997. [3] The FDA had approved five previous statin drugs—Mevacor, Zocor, Lipitor, Lescol, and Pravachol—but the excitement over Baycol was short-lived.

In December of 1999, less than two years after its release, Baycol presented undeniable problems when several reports of deaths due to rhabdomyolysis reached the FDA. [4] Bayer, the maker of the drug, and the FDA warned physicians to be cautious in prescribing it, advising against starting patients on the highest dose (0.8 mg) and telling them not to prescribe Baycol to patients who were already taking another cholesterol-lowering drug, Lopid. [5] There was found to be a significant drug-interaction when used together.

In spite of warnings, Baycol's circulation reached an estimated seven hundred thousand patients in its last twelve months on the market.

Patients taking the higher dose and those taking both Baycol and Lopid seemed to be even more susceptible to developing the muscle-destroying disease. Reports of deaths continued, and the FDA was forced to ask Bayer to take Baycol off the market in August, 2001.[6] More than fifty deaths were reported worldwide, and 1,100 reports of suspected cases of rhabdomyolysis were believed to be an adverse drug reaction to Baycol.[7]

Known Inherent Risk

According to James Cleeman, director of the National Cholesterol Education Program, "Most of the patients who were on Baycol will [instead] be placed on one of the other five 'statin' drugs still on the market. Incidentally, these drugs have also been linked to the same rare muscle weakness, known as *myositis*, which occurs in about 1 in 1,000 'statin' users. This condition occasionally progresses to rhabdomyolysis."[8]

As Cleeman explained, the development of rhabdomyolysis has become an undeniable potential risk with *all* statin drugs, even though the exact number of cases is not known due to the FDA's limited post-market surveillance. The majority of physicians are familiar with the muscle aches that frequently accompany these medications; however, most physicians are not giving adequate warnings and precautions in the use of the statin drugs they are prescribing at record levels.

> Most physicians are not giving adequate warnings and precautions in the use of the statin drugs they are prescribing at record levels.

Within the United States, the medical watchdog organization, Public Citizens' Health Research Group, petitioned the FDA to put a clearly visible warning or even a "black box" warning on all statin drugs because of the potential danger they *all* carry in causing rhabdomyolysis. The group also urged drug companies and the FDA to require an educational brochure explaining the risks of these drugs for every patient prescribed them.[9] As of this time of the publication of this book, the FDA hadn't taken any action.

Since the late 1980s, the Public Citizens' Health Research Group claims it has found eighty-one reports of deaths from rhabdomyolysis linked to statin drugs, not including the ones reported on Baycol. [10]

Statin drugs have also been known to cause liver damage. The FDA recommends that physicians get a baseline liver function on every patient they start on these drugs, then conduct follow-up liver function tests at six weeks, twelve weeks, and periodically thereafter. [11]

Again, when we discuss the potential risks drugs may create, physicians are at fault for not heeding warnings; and patients, for the most part, are not questioning their doctors, especially in situations like Bob's.

The Baycol story illustrates the important truth that all statin drugs can cause rhabdomyolysis and liver damage. But this chapter's message is broader still: we must learn to live with the continuing reality of a clear and present danger of our broader drug culture. The fact remains that even though one dangerous drug has been removed from the market, all drugs remaining still have an inherent risk. Have you ever carefully weighed the risks versus the benefits of your medication? Knowing the potential danger of any of the medications you are taking is critical and may be lifesaving. This is even true for the statin drugs that remain on the market; however, their risk is significantly lower than was the risk of taking Baycol. If the doctor or patient recognizes these adverse drug reactions soon enough, they are usually totally reversible.

I cannot tell you how many patients I've had to take off statin drugs after they developed muscle aches. These side effects are common, and I warn all my patients to quit taking their medication at the first sign of unusual muscle pain or weakness.

Kay's Story

Kay had always been in good health and was very conscientious about exercising and eating right. Inheriting a long family history of heart disease and high-cholesterol levels, she was careful to have routine check-ups. Then her family doctor informed her that medication was her only option for getting her cholesterol down into a safer range.

Kay's doctor had warned her about the potential dangers of taking statin drugs, carefully detailing how she should watch for any sign of muscle pain or weakness that seemed unusual. He also checked her liver function as a baseline before he would even start her on the cholesterol-lowering drug.

Even though her cholesterol-lowering drug was working well, Kay was burdened with the high cost of the medication because her insurance wasn't covering it. When she mentioned this to her doctor, he suggested switching her to 0.8 mg of Baycol, with eight weeks' worth of free samples.

Within three weeks of starting the new drug samples, Kay noticed that her legs started cramping, especially in her calves. She thought she must have strained them and didn't pay much attention at first. But the pain steadily grew worse and began spreading upward into her back. Then she remembered her doctor's warning about the cholesterol-lowering drugs he had prescribed. Kay quit the medication immediately. Frightened, she called her doctor.

His response was an urgent one. She needed to come in that same afternoon. He realized that any of the statin drugs could cause muscle aches or weakness. He was very concerned about Kay because her symptoms had happened so fast and were more severe than he had seen before.

By the time Kay got to his office, her legs had become weak to the point that she had difficulty climbing the stairs leading into the doctor's office. Kay's doctor showed great concern but still was not exactly certain what was happening, because it was so severe. Although he was aware of the fact that Baycol could be the culprit he wanted to be sure something else was not happening. He discontinued her Baycol and felt it would be best for his patient to see a local rheumatologist right away.

The specialist ran several tests checking for hepatitis, lupus, and even Lou Gehrig's disease. The rheumatologist then noted that one of Kay's muscle enzymes (called a CPK) was significantly elevated. A muscle biopsy soon revealed that she had developed rhabdomyolysis. The rheumatologist admitted Kay and monitored her kidney function closely.

Kay was one of the fortunate ones who never got into serious trouble while taking Baycol. Because she noticed the complications early, she was soon able to leave the hospital, and her strength slowly returned as the muscle pain diminished. She cannot express enough gratitude for her physician's personal care and his quick response. He had spent just enough extra time with her to explain the potential dangers of the medications he was prescribing. In fact, both the rheumatologist and the nephrologist commented that her stopping the medication quickly probably saved her life.

Symptomatic Suspicions

Kay's story reiterates a very important point: physicians need to be more aware of the potential dangers drugs can cause. The overriding tendency is to begin working up symptoms with the intent of looking for another disease rather than first considering the likelihood that new symptoms are a reaction from a drug previously prescribed. In Kay's case, the physician wisely had her quit taking the Baycol before he started to do his workup.

> Just because the FDA decides to leave a particular drug on the market does not, by any stretch of the imagination, mean that it is safe.

Statin drugs are simply one example of the clear-and-present-danger medications available to the patient. I use them as yet another illustration that *all drugs are known to have potentially serious and life-threatening side effects.* Political pressure, media pressure, other drug choices, and pressure from the legal profession are just some of the variables determining which drugs remain and which ones are withdrawn. Just because the FDA decides to leave a particular drug on the market does not, by any stretch of the imagination, mean that it is totally safe.

Me-Too Drugs

How many drugs are too many? How many brands of drugs are truly necessary to treat a particular ailment? If there are already twenty effective nonsteroidal anti-inflammatories (NSAIDS) on the market, is there need for one more? One of the most significant shifts in drug development over the past fifteen to twenty years is to bring out a similar drug to compete with a successful drug already on the market.

A growing trend within the pharmaceutical industry comes in the form of "Me-Too" medications. When a new drug has success in the marketplace, it is protected with a patent the FDA grants it. No pharmaceutical company can market a generic form of the drug until this patent expires. Yet other drug manufacturers often rush to find *similar but chemically different* drugs in order to capture some market share of a successful drug. They then submit these medications for New Drug Applications and can receive their own patents. This allows them to compete in the open market with an already successful drug.

Me-Too drugs rarely offer considerable medical advantages over their predecessors. Therefore, the marketing strategy of a Me-Too drug usually entails convincing physicians that this drug is just as good as its predecessor, except:

- it costs less.
- it is easier to swallow.
- it truly lasts twenty-four hours with once-a-day dosage.
- it is conveniently packaged.
- it has fewer side effects.
- the salesperson is nicer than the competition's.
- the salesperson brings nicer lunches or prettier gifts.
- patients see it advertised more on TV.

Good examples of Me-Too drugs appear in the blood-pressure medication market. There is a group of ACE inhibitors prescribed for high blood pressure and heart failure. Some of the first ACE inhibitors were Capoten (captopril) and Vasotec (enalapril). Over the next few years, Monopril (fosinopril), Lotensin (benazepril), Prinivil (lisinopril), Accupril (quinapril), and Altace (ramipril) were released onto the market.

The FDA next released, for the treatment of high blood pressure, a new family of similar drugs: angiotensin II antagonists (known as ARBs).

The first drug in this class of drugs was Cozaar (losartan). It was not any more effective than the ACE inhibitors as far as lowering blood pressure, but it had the advantage of producing less coughing, a common side effect of ACE inhibitors. Other angiotensin II antagonists then hit the marketplace, like Diovan, Avapro, Atacand, Benicar, Teveten, and Micardis. More will release even before this book reaches bookstores.

You get the picture. Please know that just because a similar drug on the market has been safe and effective, a Me-Too drug may yet have problems. Baycol is a perfect example of this principal. The FDA released it well after Mevacor and several of the other statin drugs, but it was certainly much more hazardous. It is also important to remember that Me-Too drugs always come onto the market promising glowing reports and minimal side effects. You know why: no one fully knows all the problems with new drugs.

The following table lists drugs that the FDA has removed from the marketplace. It illustrates when the FDA first approved the drug and when it forced its withdrawal. (Remember—physicians and patients must assess every drug on its own merits and not because of the class of drugs it falls into. Many brands still remain in the market category of medications that the FDA has withdrawn.)

Drugs Approved and Later Removed from the Market			
Drug Name	Year New Drug Application Approved	Year Withdrawn in United States	Months on Market
Omniflox	1992	1992	4
Redux	1996	1997	16
Pondimin	1973	1997	290
Seldane	1985	1998	152
Posicor	1997	1998	11
Duract	1997	1999	11
Raxar	1997	2000	24
Rezulin	1997	2000	38
Propulsid	1993	2000	66
Baycol	1997	2001	48

The Rest of the Story

I have focused much of this book on medications that the FDA has removed from the market. Once a drug has finally been withdrawn, its acute problems are openly admitted to the public and we learn "the rest of the story." But while a drug is still on the market, few really know or are able to discuss all of the potential problems for fear of legal or economic consequences. This in part is due to the fact that drugs are considered innocent until proven guilty. Even when they are strongly incriminated by the medical literature or FDA, many times these drugs are simply removed from the marketplace voluntarily by the pharmaceutical company. So what does this mean for all the drugs that are presently available?

> The denial and misinformation regarding drugs on the market today is concerning.

The denial and misinformation regarding drugs on the market today is concerning. It is imperative to understand that every single drug has a history and developing story behind it and patients and physicians are reporting possible severe adverse reactions to the FDA all of the time. I have mentioned that it is extremely unusual for the FDA to reverse its prior decision of drug approval. Be assured, the evidence against a particular drug has to be *overwhelming* for the FDA to make that decision and actually remove a drug from the market. Most often, physicians do not learn of the evolving problems with a particular medication until its manufacturer issues a warning or takes the drug off the market. Therefore, as I've said before: both physicians and patients need to raise their antennae high to the ongoing danger of drugs on the market.

> Early recognition of an adverse drug reaction is your best safeguard against sustaining a serious or life-threatening injury.

Prescribed medication should be the number-one suspect when new symptoms arise. Plainly spoken, the sooner you stop taking a drug that is causing a serious reaction, the better your chances of recovering—Kay's story is a perfect example. Early recognition of an adverse drug reaction is your best safeguard against sustaining a serious or life-threatening injury.

When patients make themselves aware of the potential dangers of a particular drug, they will be apt to suspect a drug reaction when something unusual arises, and they can stop the detrimental effects of an adverse drug reaction even sooner. All medications—new or old— present a "clear and present danger." Knowing everything about the drugs you are presently taking or that your doctor has prescribed is essential to your health. We must live and choose wisely each day, knowing well the presiding hazards of medication.

CHAPTER EIGHT

Mix and Match: Drug Interactions

BESIDES THE FACT THAT MANY POSSIBLE SERIOUS ADVERSE SIDE effects of a new drug are yet unknown, no one can fully predict how a particular drug will interact with other drugs. Yet few realize the full implications of taking different drugs together. The dangers of drug interactions are unprecedented as a result of the thousands of mixes and matches available with prescription drugs, over-the-counter drugs, and herbal therapies. In fact, drug interactions actually pose a much more serious threat than even the unknown side effects of newly released drugs.

The combined use of fenfluramine and phentermine for weight loss is a classic illustration of an unexpected deadly drug interaction. These drugs rapidly became known as the famous "Fen-Phen" combination that gained great popularity as a weight-loss program in the mid-1990s. It is also another tragic example of physicians' "off-label" use of medications. (The FDA approved the prescription appetite suppressant phentermine for single-drug, short-term—"a few weeks"—treatment for obesity in 1959. And in 1973 the FDA also approved fenfluramine as a single drug, with short-term use as a prescription appetite suppressant.) [1]

Patients literally flocked into my office wanting to be placed on the Fen-Phen drug program for weight loss. They all claimed to have friends or family members who had successfully lost weight using these drugs, and they wanted to try them, too. Call me old-fashioned, but I've never been a fan of using diet pills as an effective means of weight management. When I'd inform my patients about studies that showed 98 percent of the patients who took Fen-Phen gained back all of the weight they lost (and usually more), they insisted that everyone they knew was *staying on* the medication and keeping the weight off.

> Drug interactions actually pose a much more serious threat than even the unknown side effects of newly released drugs.

Shaking my head, I'd say, "So you're telling me that you want to stay on these drugs for the rest of your life?" To my disbelief the response was usually an emphatic "Yes! I will do anything to lose excess weight and keep it off."

It's difficult to communicate here the pressure some of my patients applied to make me prescribe these two medications for weight loss. Several told me straight out that if I would not prescribe Fen-Phen, they would find another physician who would. Of course, there were physicians who would prescribe this new combo, and they were not hard to find. In the months to come, my "old-fashioned" stubborn attitude saved me much personal grief, though many others were not so fortunate.

Susan's Story

Susan, a beautiful librarian, loved the outdoors and a great book. For twenty-four years the chivalrous romances of storybook characters and the crashing waves of the beach stole her heart. Being a little dreamy, she never seemed to take notice of available young men; that is, until the day she met Dan, a stunning athlete who was kind and interesting. He stopped her dead in her tracks, and her shy, bright outlook on life intrigued him as well. After their first meeting, they dated almost a year, spending most of their free time talking and reading at the beach or playing volleyball. Plans were soon in the making for an autumn wedding.

Dan never put any pressure on Susan about her size, but when she was around him and their beach friends, she constantly felt overweight and desperately wanted to lose a few pounds before the wedding. She had been trying to diet on her own, but even with the rigors of outdoor sports, she could not seem to budge those unwanted pounds.

Susan didn't know where to turn One day she shared her dilemma with a coworker at the library. On their lunch break, Jane excitedly shared how she had lost twenty-five pounds over the past two months while taking a new combination of diet pills prescribed by her doctor. This certainly got Susan's attention! In fact, it sounded too good to be true. But Jane said that two other friends were also using the drug combination called Fen-Phen and were having incredible results. Susan could hardly wait to get an appointment with Jane's doctor.

Susan saw the doctor a week later and explained that she hoped to lose twelve to fifteen pounds before her wedding. She told him that she had been trying to diet, and even though she exercised every day, she was having no success. Without hesitation, the doctor wrote a prescription for Fen-Phen and allowed six refills. He didn't give any warnings about possible side effects of the medication. Instead, his only instructions were to see him again in two months so he could monitor how she was doing. Susan started her medication that day. With renewed excitement, she started shopping for her wedding dress.

Just as she had hoped, fourteen pounds did disappear, and her bridal gown fit perfectly on the wedding day. Dan and Susan were married on September 15, 1996. After a classic storybook wedding, they departed for their honeymoon in Hawaii. Susan took her medication along because she didn't want to gain back any weight; after all, she was receiving so many wonderful compliments, and her doctor hadn't given any indication that she should do otherwise. At her two-month follow-up visit, he had simply documented her weight loss to be sure she was doing fine with the medication.

On their honeymoon, the newlyweds avoided tourist traps and opted instead for outdoor activities like paddling out in the famous North Shore surf and hiking nature trails on Kauai. The first day was incredible, but Susan began to feel like she was really out of shape. Finding herself short of breath the next day on even some of the easiest trails, she had to stop to rest frequently. Susan felt silly because Dan was so eager to keep a steady pace; she thought, *Maybe it's just fatigue from all the wedding stress.*

After returning home, the new bride felt a little better. She returned to work in the library, but even shelving books seemed like a workout. Taking drugs concerned Susan, so she figured she would continue taking Fen-Phen for only seven months, until the refills ran out. She hoped she could then keep her weight off with her own diet and exercise plan.

Within two months' time after her prescription ended, however, she started to gain weight again, and a sense of panic began to set in when her clothes started fitting too snugly. Susan did not want to be one of those wives who looked as if she was letting herself go after she got "hitched." Dan had been so proud of her.

I've just got to raise my metabolism, she thought. She pressed on while trying to cut back on calories. During an aerobic class, Susan was embarrassed and really worried when she got winded early in warmups and had to quit the exercise just to catch her breath. Something was not right. She decided right then to go back to her own doctor rather than seeing Jane's again.

Susan's personal physician checked her thoroughly and noted that Susan had a heart murmur that she had never detected before. It was a significant murmur and she could not have missed it in previous exams. With a look of surprise, the doctor asked if Susan had been sick or developed a fever during the past year. She replied she had been fine and had not even had a sore throat. *But,* she thought, *I should at least tell her about the other doctor last summer and the diet pills.* The young patient almost chickened out but instead told her doctor the whole truth—that she had been taking the popular Fen-Phen combination.

She explained how she went to Jane's doctor because she was afraid her primary physician would have refused to prescribe it, knowing she needed to lose only fifteen pounds. The physician nodded in agreement. Then she said, "My concern now, Susan, is that the Mayo Clinic has just released a study detailing how many patients who have taken this Fen-Phen medication are now suffering heart valve complications."

The doctor immediately ordered an echocardiogram and referred Susan to a local cardiologist. Susan was terrified and called Dan to ask if he would come for the consultation. The cardiologist quietly explained to them that major damage had occurred to several heart valves, with the worst damage done to her mitral valve. No longer able to close properly, it was causing significant leaking. If this was not bad enough news, the cardiologist went on to explain that Susan's shortness of breath came as a result of her having developed primary pulmonary hypertension, for which there is no surgical procedure. He explained that this happens when the blood pressure in the arteries supplying blood to the lungs has elevated.

Susan began treatment with several different medications and was advised not to do any activity other than light walking, and even then to be very careful about hills or steps. After searching the Internet and medical textbooks about her disease, she realized that her life expectancy was not likely to exceed two to three years. Anger and frustration grew as her health began to decline. The young couple decided to sue the makers of Fen-Phen in an attempt to help defray some of the overwhelming medical costs. They won an undisclosed settlement from the company a year later.

Susan's death four years following her initial prescription of Fen-Phen was attributed to complications of pulmonary hypertension. Dan watched his beautiful young bride die after spending her brief marriage either in the hospital or sick in bed. Devastated, he spent long hours remembering how his bride had been so full of life when they had first met, before her life and dreams had been snatched away. Sadness overwhelmed him, knowing that all of her suffering and needless death could have been avoided. None of this had to happen, if only . . . if only.

––––––

The damage the dangerous combination Fen-Phen wrought on one young woman's heart was multiplied over and over again. On July 8,

1997, the Mayo Clinic reported twenty-four cases of significant heart-valve damage in women who had taken the drug combination for weight loss.[2] The findings so concerned researchers that they broke the normal confidentiality of medical studies prior to publishing in order to warn officials at the FDA. The FDA immediately sent out seven hundred thousand warning letters to physicians and other health-care providers. [3]

The FDA soon received spontaneous reports of an additional 140 cases of valvular damage in patients using Fen-Phen and another new drug, dexfenfluramine (Redux).[4] Twenty-seven of these patients required cardiac valve-replacement surgery. [5] The FDA also received echocardiographic reports from five independent institutions and clinics. The actual prevalence of valvular disease in patients taking Fen-Phen for greater than six months was approximately 33 percent, or one-third, of the patients. Many of these patients also developed primary pulmonary hypertension, like Susan.[6] Can you imagine?

It was shocking to learn that one-third of the patients who took Fen-Phen for a period of at least six months had serious heart valve damage, many of whom required open-heart surgery to replace the damaged valve(s). The frequency of valve damage in patients who took Fen-Phen for less than three months was 22 percent. The FDA estimated that three to four million Americans had taken Fen-Phen for longer than three months since 1995 for weight loss.[7]

The FDA never intended that patients use these drugs in combination and had never approved them for long-term use. Though a minority of the medical reports advocated remaining on this drug combination indefinitely, most reports suggested that people stay on the drug regimen no longer than three to six months. [8]

Remarkably, fenfluramine had been on the market for twenty-four years without notable complications. It wasn't until several reports in the medical literature highlighted patients' remarkable weight loss after taking fenfluramine and phentermine in tandem that the combination became popular almost overnight.

The interaction between the drugs was unmistakable, illustrating one of the major problems with off-label use—the inherent risk of drug interactions. Remember, *off-label use* refers to when health-care providers prescribe drugs for diseases or in ways the FDA has not studied or approved. Even though both drugs had been around for years, they had never been used together. Since both were readily available in the pharmacies, physicians simply had to write two different prescriptions, which they and their patients believed were perfectly safe.

Real-Life Scenarios

Clinical trials do not model real-life scenarios. Though they may be representative to a certain degree of a population at large, Chapter 2 briefly describes how these experiments are strategically designed and carefully controlled. Investigators tend to choose the healthiest subjects possible for their clinical trials, enabling pharmaceutical companies the best chance to find needed evidence the drug is effective in treating a specific ailment with as few side effects as possible.

It is especially important to remember that when the FDA is evaluating a drug during the approval process, clinical trials involve either healthy subjects or patients without additional problems or diseases other than the one being studied. Furthermore, these selected populations of people are not usually taking any drugs other than the one being studied. This is obviously not what happens in reality.

Real-life situations are filled with complicated dynamics, perhaps the most important one being that most patients suffer from a number of simultaneous illnesses and seek treatment from a variety of specialists. How many medical specialists do you see each year? If you have parents living, how many do they have? In an era of specialized medical care, patients see a host of unrelated specialists that may include family practitioners, rheumatologists, cardiologists, dermatologists, pulmonologists, and even neurologists.

Typically, each specialist prescribes at least two or three different drugs, sometimes without being entirely aware of what other physicians may be prescribing the same patient. This is definitely beyond the scope of clinical trials. Why do we feel safe with a new medication that investigators have tested only on relatively healthy subjects? On one hand we have the results of carefully recorded clinical trial conditions with healthy subjects—an ideal and certainly an unrealistic scenario—and on the other, we have patients suffering with complicated health issues seeing several different specialists, each prescribing medications. This is a real-life scenario.

Americans are consuming medications of all shapes and sizes in record amounts. In 1997 alone, pharmacies filled an estimated 2.35 billion prescriptions. This means each person receives an average of 11.6 prescriptions per year. Most patients are taking two or more different drugs, and many patients are taking as many as eight to ten different drugs at the same time.[9] Believe it or not, I know several patients who are taking as many as twenty-five to thirty different drugs daily!

> It is truly impossible to know precisely how a drug will interact in a patient who is on *several different* drugs at the same time.

Granted, it may be possible to anticipate how *two* drugs may interact with one another. You might even be able to predict how a drug will react when coupled with *two* other drugs. But it is truly impossible to know precisely how a drug will interact in a patient who is on *several different* drugs at the same time. What are the odds of winning a jackpot lottery? The odds of knowing the outcome of mixing numerous drugs are the same.

New drugs are especially dangerous in this situation. Once the FDA has released a drug and the major marketing blitz immediately kicks in, physicians write millions of prescriptions for a new medication within its first few months on the market. Patients who are much more ill than those in the premarket clinical trials will use these drugs, and they're probably taking many more prescription drugs as well.

Premarketing clinical trials can never fully duplicate or evaluate real life. It follows then that the FDA cannot possibly determine the results of mixing and matching drugs until you, the patient, discover them. Before you add a new drug to your regimen, take a moment to read how drugs interact and break down simultaneously within the liver (otherwise known as drug metabolism).

Drug Metabolism

The human body has a tremendous ability to detoxify and rid itself of many different toxic substances (including medications), primarily through the liver and kidneys. Due to the great number of drugs patients are now consuming, however, serious and life-threatening problems continue to occur more readily. Let me explain why.

Because drugs are synthetic (not natural), they are basically toxic substances to the body. Our liver is the center for detoxifying many of these drugs through its many different enzyme systems. It breaks down the drugs into intermediate by-products and eventually eliminates them from the body. Each drug primarily utilizes one specific enzyme system to break it down. One of the most commonly used enzyme systems for this process is called the *cytochrome P450 system*.

> The FDA cannot possibly determine the results of mixing and matching drugs until you, the patient, discover them.

Perhaps the easiest way to understand the challenges the liver has in the breakdown of combined drugs is to imagine your five-year-old pouring a pound of sugar through a funnel with an opening one centimeter in diameter. Or perhaps you can relate more fully to driving on a five-lane freeway at rush hour only to discover a flashing arrow alerting you and thousands of other drivers that, due to construction, the freeway is about to narrow to one lane. Can you relate? Either you will have sticky sugar all over the kitchen counters and floor or you are in one of the cars lined up for miles waiting to merge, wishing you had chosen a side street before getting sandwiched into a long wait.

Bottlenecking occurs in our livers, too. When a person takes a variety of drugs, each utilizing different enzyme systems within the liver (like different routes through the city), seldom do complications occur. But when he is taking two or more drugs requiring the same enzyme system within the liver to metabolize and eliminate the drugs from the body, blood levels of the drugs may climb to dangerous levels.

During the metabolism of a particular drug, another serious concern may also arise. Like smog that forms in a thick, orange haze while cars sit idle on the freeway, a drug may actually become even more toxic in its intermediate by-products (called *toxic metabolites*) before being eliminated from the body. In other words, the liver may need to change a drug chemically several different times into a product that the body can excrete. The products created by this process may pose more danger than the drug itself, especially if there is a backup in the liver slowing down this entire process.

Over the years, both the FDA and physicians have become more and more aware of the dangers that drug metabolism presents. Again, during premarketing clinical trials, the drug under scrutiny may indeed test safe. But in a real-life scenario when different drugs must compete for a particular enzyme system, not only might the drug levels themselves soar to dangerous levels, but toxic metabolites may also increase significantly. The release of Posicor, a calcium channel blocker primarily used for hypertension, clearly illustrates this situation.

Posicor

Posicor was the tenth calcium channel blocker, a blood pressure medication that the FDA approved, even after a number of advisory members showed alarm during premarketing clinical trials when a seventy-year-old man suffered sudden death (remember the Me-Too drug phenomenon). Senior FDA officials were also concerned when 142 other sudden deaths were reported in an ongoing study using Posicor in patients with congestive heart failure.[10]

The FDA had to make a choice. Would it approve Posicor, or wait another year or more until it knew all of the study details? In spite of the fact that several members didn't find the drug offering any unique quality not already available on the market, the committee voted five to three in favor of approving the drug for immediate release.[11]

Consistent with the FDA's new pattern of aggressive approval since the legislative change in 1992, the agency released Posicor with a warning to physicians in "tiny" print on the drug's information label.[12] It advised doctors against prescribing the medicine in combination with *twenty-five* other drugs and even in combination with the eating of grapefruit (which also uses the cytochrome P450 system). You may be able to guess why: Posicor used the cytochrome P450 enzyme system to metabolize and eliminate itself from the body, and the FDA knew there were already numerous other drugs on the market that also used this same enzyme system.

A list of medications that utilize the cytochrome P450 enzyme system in metabolism appears in Table 1 on the following page.

Another grave concern with Posicor arose when patients experienced acute lowering of their heart rates as blood levels of the drug increased. In other words, very little margin of error existed between the therapeutic blood levels of the drug and the toxic levels, which could cause dangerously low heart rates to occur. In addition, when patients took Posicor with cholesterol-lowering drugs (like the statin drugs I discussed in the last chapter, common for patients who have high blood pressure), several patients experienced even more serious slowing of their heart rates.[13]

The drug company agreed to change its label to include a warning against the use of Posicor with several cholesterol-lowering drugs. In spite of changes in the label, in came more and more reports relating the new medication to possible deaths. On June 8, 1998, the pharmaceutical company withdrew Posicor from the market.[14]

Several FDA advisory members believed the agency should never have approved it in the first place. Janet Woodcock of the FDA, however, argued that the problems that "sunk" Posicor were unexpected and that the FDA anticipated better compliance with the advice in the drug's label.[15] What do you think?

Drugs That Interact with Coumadin

Doctors prescribe Coumadin, a fairly common blood-thinning drug, frequently to folks in the elderly population to prevent the formation of unwanted blood clots and to prevent strokes. Typically, patients who take Coumadin are on several other medications and many over-the-counter

Table 1

Drugs That Use the Cytochrome P450 System

Aciphex	Darvocet	Lipitor	Prozac
Actos	Detrol	Lopid	Remeron
Advair	Diabeta	Lopressor	Risperdal
Amaryl	Diflucan	Luvox	Singulair
Ambien	Dilantin	Mevacor	Soma
Amitriptyline	Effexor	Micronase	Sporanox
Anaprox	Erythromycin	Naproxen	Tegretol
Avandia	Feldene	Nexium	Trazadone
Avapro	Flagyl	Norvasc	Tricor
Biaxin	Flonase	Oxycodone	Ultram
Cardizem	Flovent	Paxil	Valium
Celebrex	Glucotrol	Phenergan	Viagra
Celexa	Grapefruit	Plavix	Voltaren
Cipro	Hydrocodone	Plendil	Wellbutrin
Claritin	Ibuprofen	Prednisone	Xanax
Codeine	Inderal	Prevacid	Zocor
Cordarone	Indocin	Prilosec	Zoloft
Coreg	Isoptin	Procardia	Zyprexa
Coumadin	Klonopin	Propoxophene	
Cozaar	Lescol	Protonix	

medications such as aspirin, Aleve, Motrin, and Tylenol, any of which can interact with this drug.

Doctors must frequently check protimes (a blood test that determines how thin the blood is) in patients who are taking Coumadin. Below you will find a partial list of substances that interact with this medication.

(See Table 2, Drugs That Interact with Coumadin on the following page.)

Foods that interfere with Coumadin include foods rich in vitamin K, such as asparagus, bacon, beef liver, cabbage, fish, cauliflower, and green, leafy vegetables.

Herbal medicines to avoid while taking Coumadin are angelica root, anise, borage-seed oil, devil's claw, papain, ginseng, ginger, ginkgo, horse chestnut, alfalfa, red clover, clove oil, feverfew, passionflower herb, salvia root (danshen), willow bark, cinchona bark, turmeric, garlic, coquinone, and dong quai.

Occasionally patients on Coumadin suffer a serious adverse drug reaction, possibly even a life-threatening bleed. How often does your doctor or pharmacist give you an entire list of drugs to avoid if you are taking this medication?

Table 2

Drugs That Interact with Coumadin (warfarin)

The following drugs may *increase* the effects of Coumadin (warfarin):

abciximab (Reopro)
acarbose (Precose)
acetaminophen (Tylenol, especially if more than 2,275 mg per week is taken)
allopurinol (Zyloprim)
alteplase (Activase) and is contraindicated if the prothrombin time is more than 15 seconds
amiodarone (Cordarone)
amprenavir (Agenerase)
androgens
aspirin and some other NSAIDS
azithromycin (Zithromax)
bismuth subsalicylate (Pepto Bismol)
some calcium channel blockers (various) have been associated with an increased risk of stomach and intestine (gastrointestinal) hemorrhage. This risk may be exacerbated by warfarin use.
carbamozepine (Tegretol)
cephalosporins
choral hydrate (Noctec)
chloramphenicol (Chloromycetin)
cimetidine (Tagamet)
ciprofloxacin and other quinolone antibiotics
disopyramide (Norpace)
disulfiram (Antabuse)
enoxaparin (Lovenox)
erythromycin (various)
felbamate (Felbatol)
fluconazole (Diflucan)
fluoxetine (Prozac)
fluvastatin (Lescol) and perhaps similar drugs
fluvoxamine (Luvox)
fosphenytoin (Cerebyx) or phenytoin (Dilantin)
gemfibrozil (Lopid)
glucagon
heparin (various)
HMG CoA-reductase inhibitors (Zocor, Mevacor, Lipitor, Pravachol, Lescol)
influenza vaccine (various)
isohaizid (INH)
itraconazole (Sporanox)
ketoconazole (Nizoral)
mesna (Mesnex)
methyltestosterone (any 17-alkylated androgen)
metronidazole (Flagyl)
miconazole (Monistat)
minocycline
nonsteroidal anti-inflammatory drugs

omeprazole (Prilosec)
orlistat (Xenical)
paroxetine (Paxil)
pravastatin (Pravachol)
propafenone (Rythmol)
propranolol (Inderal)
propoxyphene (various)
quinidine (Quinaglute)
quetiapine (Seroquel)
rantidine (Zantac)
ritonavir (Norvir) and perhaps other protease inhibitors
salicylates (aspirin, etc.)
sertraline (Zoloft)
simvastatin (Zocor)
streptokinase
sulfinpyrazone (Anturane)
sulfonamides
tamoxifen (Nolvadex)
tamsulosin (Flomax)
terbinafine (Lamisil)
testosterone (various)
tetracyclines
thyroid hormones (various)
thrombolytic drugs (such as ateplase)
tramadol (Ultram)
trastuzumab (Herceptin)
tricyclic antidepressants
vancomycim (Vancoled)
vitamin E
zafirlukast (Accolate)
zileuton (Zyflo)
zotepine (Nipolept)

The following drugs may *decrease* the effects of Coumadin (warfarin):

antithyroid agents (various) by decreasing prior high rates of clotting metabolism
azathioprine (Imuran)
barbiturates
birth control pills (oral contraceptives)
carbamazepine (Tegretol)
chlordiazepoxide (Librium)
cholestyramine (Questran)
estrogens (various)
ethchlorvynol (Placidyl)
glutethimide (Doriden)
griseofulvin (Gris-PEG)
phenobarbital (various)
vitamin K

Similar Side Effects

Would you think twice if your physician prescribed you Seldane, the first non-sedating antihistamine, along with Erythromycin for an upper respiratory infection? Most patients wouldn't. The combination seems to be a logical one. But a serious incident occurred, and it occurred frequently, with many devastating results.

Seldane illustrates another important aspect of drug interactions. This drug's potential danger came not from interactions due to enzyme systems bottlenecking during metabolism, but as a result of the *actual pharmaceutical effect of the drug itself.* Some drugs that are known to have side effects don't pose much of a threat when taken alone. But when a patient takes them along with other medications with similar side effects, the combination may prove life-threatening. Such was the case with Seldane.

When patients used Seldane by itself, problems rarely occurred. When, on the other hand, a patient combined it with the common antibiotic Erythromycin, or the antifungal drug Nizoral (ketoconazol), a patient could develop a cardiac arrest.[16]

A known effect of the drug is that it prolonged the QT interval, the conduction of electrical currents through the heart. (See Chapter 6.) When investigators studied Seldane in preclinical controlled studies, they reported no problems. Again, this drug was primarily used alone in all of the preliminary trials. In the real world, however, Seldane was frequently prescribed with Erythromycin (patients who had allergies would frequently get upper respiratory infections or bronchitis) and occasionally Nizoral. Both are drugs that also cause prolongation of the QT interval—in which case the effects were exaggerated and proved deadly.[17] On the market for twelve years before the FDA finally withdrew it, this non-sedating antihistamine proved to be the culprit in many deaths.

———

Indisputably, drug interactions create extremely complex and unpredictable difficulties. Voluminous textbooks, intricate charts, and software have been written on the subject in an attempt to make sense of all the known drawbacks of these potentially dangerous situations. Physicians can only hope to understand the most common and basic problems of drug interactions.

Clinical trials can never provide a true reflection of real-life scenarios in which people are suffering from and being treated simultaneously for several illnesses at a time. Remember, physicians prescribe new drugs most often to patients who are very ill and are already taking several other drugs. Not only can each individual drug cause a serious adverse reaction, but as more and more drugs are added, the risk of adverse drug reactions goes up exponentially (1 plus 1 does not equal 2, but rather 8 or 10).

CHAPTER NINE

Polydoc

CHAMBERLAIN, A SMALL TOWN OF THREE THOUSAND LOCATED on the Missouri River in the middle of South Dakota, was the place of my beginnings. Life was hard but good. If you got sick in Chamberlain you drove downtown to the community hospital where you made one of two choices: you either visited Dr. Holland or Dr. Binder. My family chose Dr. Holland.

Dr. Holland knew just about everybody in town, but he *knew* my family not only by name, but "from one end to the other." He treated all my strep throats, sutured my lacerations, repaired my hernia when I was thirteen, and hospitalized me for three weeks when I developed Guillain-Barré syndrome at age sixteen. If I close my eyes, I can still smell his office to this day.

Dr. Holland was a fixture in Chamberlain. He attended every basketball and football game without ever sitting down. Instead he always stood by the door. I'm sure he did this in case he had to make a quick exit for the hospital. I grew up with all of his children and even dated his daughter. His life was one I deeply admired. How impressed I was to see him in his office late at night, reading the latest medical journals, when I brought his daughter home from a date.

Doc Holland, my family physician with large, warm hands and an engaging smile, was the only doctor I saw until I went to college. In fact, his influence is still far-reaching in my life. Not only am I writing about him in admiration forty years later, but he played an important role in convincing me to pursue a career in medicine. I realize now the lasting impact he made by always ensuring time for a friendly, personal conversation in spite of his busy schedule.

Between 80 and 85 percent of all physicians in America are specialists.

How times have changed! Now between 80 and 85 percent of all physicians in America are specialists. Medicine is a fascinating and overwhelming career. Each year researchers make remarkable discoveries in every capacity, demanding focused attention. One simply cannot begin to learn all there is to know about every aspect of medicine. Specialists are not only important but essential in the complete and sophisticated care patients often require.

But there is a trade-off. Specialists can spend only limited amounts of time with each of their patients—perhaps never becoming familiar with the patients' families. I believe this is one of the reasons I chose to become a family physician. Instead of joining the shift toward specialization, I wanted to offer the personalized care that Dr. Holland gave me. Besides, I liked the variety that family practice offered.

On one hand, I enjoyed each specialty presented during my training, and I grew to admire the scientific breakthroughs and treatments offered through specialized care. On the other hand, my appreciation grew for Dr. Holland, knowing he delivered me, took care of all aspects of my health, did my surgery, took care of my parents, and was a personal friend. Being involved in my patients' lives was especially important to me and therefore, I made my choice.

When I started my practice in Rapid City, South Dakota, in 1972, most of the seventy-five active doctors at that time were primary-care physicians. Over the next few years, many visionaries helped Rapid City grow into a major medical center for western South Dakota, Wyoming, and Nebraska. I had the privilege of knowing many of these great people—but one doctor in particular not only understood the importance that specialty care had to offer patients, he was willing to do whatever it took to make his vision a reality.

Dr. Myron Jerde was one of the general internists practicing in Rapid City when I first arrived. I had great respect for him. When I first met Dr. Jerde, he ran the pulmonary lab, the dialysis unit, and performed all GI endoscopy work, in addition to being an excellent and busy general internist.

With confidence both in his work and in the growing needs of the future, he actively went out of his way to help recruit Rapid City's first pulmonologist. He graciously backed away from his own work in this field, turning all specialty pulmonary care to Dr. Bill Howard. Dr. Jerde then helped to hire an excellent gastroenterologist, Dr. Ken Vogele. Again, he strongly encouraged medical practitioners to support the new specialist to help build his practice.

Finally, he located and recruited a nephrologist to run the dialysis unit. Today, approximately 250 physicians are involved in active practice in Rapid City, South Dakota; about 75 to 80 percent of them are specialists. Our city has become a regional medical center, most likely similar to one near you.

Superspecialization

I never cease to be amazed at the growing demand for specialized care. Several years ago a friend who had recently become an orthopedic surgeon asked if I thought there would be enough work for him to start his own practice in Rapid City. After conferring with me and several other physicians in the area, Dr. Dave Boyer did, in fact, decide to start his practice in our city.

I remember how astonished I was when trying to schedule a patient with him about two weeks after he'd arrived; his nurse promptly informed me that it would take about six weeks to get an appointment. Dr. Boyer's group has since moved into its own large clinic. The staff includes an orthopedic surgeon specializing in joint replacement, another who does surgery primarily on the shoulder, one who specializes in back problems, and another who primarily works on feet.

This *superspecialization* is occurring in all fields of medicine. Even parts of the same organ now require specialty training. No longer are patients with eye problems going to the eye doctor or opthalmologist, but rather to a specialist on retinal disease, or a specialist in lens replacement, a neuro-opthalmologist, or a refractive eye surgeon. It wasn't long ago when specializing in the eye alone, although very important indeed, seemed to be limiting oneself.

Specialization offers many great strengths and advancements in medical technology, which would require several volumes of its own to do it justice. Instead, I'm here to ask, *How does specialized medicine affect you, the patient, when it comes to serious adverse drug reactions?*

Many patients no longer have a primary-care doctor. They "float" in a clinic made up of several specialists or see specialists located throughout their community. Specialists tend to prescribe more potent medications, usually in combination with several other medications, because these patients have more serious medical problems. Consequently, these medications carry the greatest risk of serious adverse drug reactions and interactions.

> Specialists tend to prescribe more potent medications, usually in combination with several other medications, because these patients have more serious medical problems.

Fragmented Health Care

It's very common to see patients who are consulting three or four different specialists for their medical care (nearly 50 percent of patients in the United States are seeing more than one physician[1]), and it's not uncommon to see patients who are taking anywhere between eight and twenty different drugs at the same time. For all the strengths of specialization, we must be especially aware of its latent effect—on the flip side is a fragmented system of health care.

Not only is there a tendency for each specialist to prescribe several drugs, but the communication between various specialists and between the specialists and the primary physician is not always ideal. This leads to patients taking several different drugs, which can significantly increase their risk of drug interactions, especially with the possibility of physicians not being entirely aware of all the medications the patients may be taking.

As patients develop health problems, they will most definitely see more specialists in the future. Specialty care is the medical trend of both today and tomorrow. I realize that even though I'm a family physician and promote primary care, most of the patients I see have a different attitude.

When a patient has a lung problem, he wants to see the best in the field—a pulmonologist. If he needs surgery on his prostate, he wants the surgeon who does the procedure thirty to forty times a month, not several times a year. Earaches need the care of an ear, nose, and throat specialist; rashes require a dermatologist. When a child gets a sore throat or cough, young parents want to see the "doc in the box," otherwise known as the seven-to-eleven urgent care doctor, because they don't want to take time out of a busy schedule to see their personal doctors. This is our medical system. Is it effective? Yes. Can it increase the risk of suffering an adverse drug reaction? Absolutely.

Specialized Care and Adverse Drug Events

Hospital Care

There is nothing I like to avoid more than having to be admitted to a hospital. Still, for those of us who become ill and require hospitalization, it is comforting to receive the sophisticated care that is now commonplace in a hospital setting. Skilled, well-trained nurses, technicians, x-ray techs, lab techs, and of course physicians are available to us in our time of need.

This care, however, is not exempt from the inherent risks of fragmented health care and the possibility of adverse drug reactions. Usually several different physicians see ill patients, and they are all writing orders for various medications, especially for the critically ill. These patients are usually not even aware of how many or what types of drugs they may be receiving.

In an article published in the *Journal of General Internal Medicine* titled "Incidence and Preventability of Adverse Drug Events in Hospitalized Adults," Dr. David Bates argued, "The potential for errors in the use of drugs is enormous. Nationally, the average patient receives ten different drugs during their hospitalization, and most critically ill patients receive many more; in our sample, the mean number was 38."[2]

Dr. Bates went on to state that several studies have estimated that as many as 10 to 15 percent of the patients admitted to hospitals suffer an adverse drug reaction during their stay.[3] Most of these cases we can simply attribute to the inherent risk of the medications and interactions of the drugs taken. Still, we can't deny that medication errors occur as well. Several recent studies estimate that between three and five medication errors take place per one thousand orders.[4] And the majority of these errors have the potential of a serious adverse drug event. Not only do we face the inherent risk of medications but also the additional risk of medication errors.

Dr. Bates made bold statements about how common adverse drug reactions are in hospitalized adults. With hospital personnel's great tendency toward concealing mistakes and the reluctance to report complications, spontaneous reporting reveals only a small portion of adverse drug reactions or medication errors. When quality-review nurses began to look specifically for these problems (without relying simply on spontaneous reports), claimed Bates, the incidence of adverse drug reactions and medication errors increased fiftyfold. After reviewing all of their findings, Bates concluded that the overwhelming majority of these cases were preventable.[5]

Doctors love their drugs, and I guarantee they will prescribe them. Whether it is in the hospital or an outpatient setting, you can anticipate that your doctor will prescribe medication for each and every complaint or problem. The move toward outpatient and specialty medical care undoubtedly contributes to greatly increasing one's risk of developing a serious adverse drug reaction.

Outpatient Health Care

As I mentioned in the introduction, between 1983 and 1993, the number of outpatient visits increased in the United States by 75 percent, while the number of inpatient days fell 21 percent.[6] Physicians are not admitting patients as often, nor do patients stay as long in the hospital as they once did. When I first started doing obstetrics, my patients would stay in the hospital for a minimum of five days. In my final years of doing obstetrics, however, when I would deliver a child, the mother's first question would be, "Is it a boy or a girl?" And the very next question—while she was still on the delivery table—was invariably "When can we go home?"

The move toward outpatient and specialty medical care undoubtedly contributes to greatly increasing one's risk of developing a serious adverse drug reaction.

The cost of hospital care has skyrocketed. These high costs force insured, Medicare, and private-pay patients out of the hospital much sooner than is healthy. Even heart bypass patients are going home five days after surgery. Simply stated, many patients are going home before they are ready.

This major trend in medicine has put tremendous reliance on outpatient medicine, meaning that outpatients are taking more medications, and they are not under the close supervision of medical personnel in the hospital. Physicians are prescribing stronger and more potent medications to cut the length of hospital stays or are dispersing them on an outpatient basis in attempt to keep patients from having to go to the hospital in the first place. Incidentally, medication errors that frequently lead to serious adverse reactions and deaths have greatly increased during this past decade.[7] One of the main reasons is because the health-care system is placing the heavy responsibility of self-care on patients' shoulders.

Use and Misuse of Antibiotics

One area that most health-care providers and public health officials agree about is the overuse of antibiotics. The rise of antibiotic-resistant bacteria should cause everyone alarm. Our overzealous use of antibiotics when we do not necessarily need them could quickly wipe out the great advances we've made in reducing deaths caused by bacterial infections over the past half-century. Drug resistance is a serious clinical and public-health problem in the United States and globally. The frequency of drug resistance is increasing in virtually all organisms that cause both community- and hospital-acquired infections.[8]

> Medication errors that frequently lead to serious adverse reactions and deaths have greatly increased during this past decade.

The Centers for Disease Control and Prevention (CDC) estimates that office-based physicians prescribe approximately 100 million courses of antibiotics in the United States each year.[9] Furthermore, the CDC estimates that health-care providers give more than 50 million of these courses to patients who simply have a cold or other viral infection, which antibiotics are not meant to treat—they help only with bacterial infections.[10]

In other words, half of the outpatient prescriptions physicians write are not necessary. Viruses do not respond to antibiotics, and one's own immune system will normally rid the body of this type of infection with time. Most patients will get better within three to four days, but the antibiotic usually gets the credit, even though it had nothing to do with the patient's improvement.

Resistant Bacteria: Survival of the Fittest

The development of bacterial resistance is the result of the well-known concept of survival of the fittest. If you take an antibiotic for a common cold or even a bacterial infection, you may wipe out 99 percent of the bacteria in your body that are sensitive to that particular antibiotic. Yet the 1 percent that was not sensitive to the antibiotic will replicate a new whole generation of bacteria that will be resistant to that particular antibiotic.

When penicillin was first introduced in the 1940s, it was able to cure almost every kind of infection: streptococcus, staphylococcus, pneumococcus, and even tuberculosis, gonorrhea, and syphilis. By the 1950s and 1960s, resistant strains of bacteria began to appear that penicillin did not destroy. Every year more and more antibiotics became available, but no one seemed to be worried about the resistance that was developing with almost every strain of bacteria. "Each time an antibiotic lost its effectiveness, there was another magic bullet on the pharmacist's shelf," wrote Dr. Patricia Lieberman in a paper published by the Center for Science in the Public Interest. "But now that shelf is almost empty. The development of new antibiotics has not kept up with the development of antibiotic resistance."[11]

> The rise of antibiotic-resistant bacteria should cause everyone alarm.

Major Educational Campaigns

Most people (especially physicians) now realize that viral infections do not respond to antibiotics. Unless doctors actually take cultures, however, they can't be certain whether a virus or a bacterium is causing the patient's sore throat, upper respiratory infection, or bronchitis. In response to continued antibiotic resistance, several agencies launched campaigns throughout the 1990s to promote the appropriate use of antibiotics by public health and professional organizations, including the CDC, American Academy of Pediatrics, American Academy of Family Practice, American Academy Society for Microbiology, and Alliance for the Prudent Use of Antibiotics.[12]

> The development of new antibiotics has not kept up with the development of antibiotic resistance.

A follow-up study reported in the *Journal of the American Medical Association* objectively considered whether these campaigns had been effective or not. Researchers looked at the pediatric use of antibiotics in 1999 and compared it to that of 1989, when antibiotic use was at its all-time high. Seemingly optimistic results showed the overall use of antibiotics fell more than 30 percent in the pediatric population during this time. But there was more to see. Interestingly, the report also revealed the fact that physician office visits for these infections also fell 30 percent.[13]

Conclusive evidence revealed that patients were listening and responding to the message of the campaigns and were not seeking medical advice if they felt their children had only a cold. In cases where parents sought medical advice from their physicians, however, the relative number of prescriptions written for antibiotic use remained the same.[14]

By educating the parents of young patients, we are making great strides in cutting down antibiotic misuse. Physicians, on the other hand, are not responding as well. Recent surveys of pediatricians found that parental pressure, rather than concern about legal liability, was the major reason that physicians were prescribing antibiotics.[15]

> You are indeed part of the solution—I believe the most important part.

Patients do have a positive effect on physicians' prescribing habits. First of all, if you do not show up in your doctor's office, he or she won't be able to prescribe any medication. Second, by telling your physician that you don't want an antibiotic unless he knows for certain that it is necessary, you and your family will be taking wise care and your doctor can practice better medicine. You are indeed part of the solution—I believe the most important part.

Taking Medications Properly

In a study Susanna Bedell, M.D., et al., reported in the *Archives of Internal Medicine*, patients studied took their medications improperly 75 percent of the time. Reports of the misuse of medications were highest in patients taking several different medications and in patients who were older in age. Additional research also reveals conclusive evidence that when a patient sees more than one physician, the risk of his taking medication improperly increased significantly. Bedell's study asked patients about their personal concerns about taking prescription meds. The following lists the top four:

1. Patients desired more detailed information from their physicians about how the drug they prescribed would help their symptoms and how it would react with other medications.
2. Patients felt that the information about adverse reactions their doctors gave them was often too vague. For example, the doctor may have told them to call back if they "felt blah" or "were not feeling themselves," rather than describing a specific symptom.
3. Patients often left the doctors' offices confused about how they should take their medication and the exact dose they should take. This proves to be a major concern because many patients receive free samples from their doctor when they are starting new medication. This totally eliminates any contact with a pharmacist, who might educate the patient further about the new prescription.
4. The majority of patients focused on the problem of having multiple physicians. When they experienced complications with their medications or instructions, access to their specialist was very limited. Many reported that their primary-care physician made prescription changes without first consulting the specialist who had originally written the script. [16]

Is the Doctor In?

If you develop a problem with your medication, how easy is it to see or consult your specialist? Do you have trouble getting access to your physician when you would like? I'm not talking about waiting too long in a doctor's waiting room. I'm referring to when you are having a medical problem—can you see your physician quickly or does it take a few days or even weeks? I anticipate your answer is generally, "It takes a while and a lot of determination." It's not easy. I know, because my patients frequently consult me in situations like these. This is a major concern when it comes to adverse drug reactions. Let me explain by an example.

A patient (let's call her Jane) will tell me that her cardiologist just prescribed a drug (let's say, Betapace) for an irregular heart rhythm. Jane will then admit that Betapace is making her feel horrible—that she's been tired and fatigued since starting this particular medication. My first question is whether she's tried to reschedule another appointment with her cardiologist. Her answer will most likely be, "Yes, but I can't get in for another three weeks." I usually then hear how my patient spoke with the cardiologist's nurse, who told her to stay on the medication until she could see the doctor.

Now the scenario has become my problem. With some medications I feel comfortable telling the patient to simply quit taking the dosage until he is able to see the specialist. But many times patients need to switch immediately to a different medication to continue treating a current problem. In this case, I first make an attempt to contact the cardiologist or specialist personally by phone, but this can be difficult even for me at times. The specialist may be in the coronary catheter lab or the intensive-care unit at the hospital. He may not be on call. If I can catch the physician outside the office, he may not remember details about the patient or why he started the medication in the first place. Sometimes I can help, but in many instances the process is extremely frustrating.

Access to your physician is critical when it comes to drug reactions. Physicians are notoriously busy people, and it can be incredibly difficult to schedule a referral patient with a particular specialist. Family physicians, pediatricians, internists, and gynecologists are not exempt either. I cannot imagine how some of my patients deal with this on a regular basis.

Office nurses frequently have to make difficult decisions about patient care too. I am amazed at some of the decisions and comments they make to patients while trying to fulfill their role in protecting their doctors. What if the patient doesn't have a primary doctor whom he can call as a backup? Patients are unfortunately often left out in the cold or directed to go straight to an emergency room.

The medical community's ability to clearly and concisely communicate patient data on a timely basis is the issue at hand. Specialization and fragmented health care make up-to-date communication mandatory. In many ways the system has gone wrong because patients are falling through its cracks. Adverse drug reactions often result from incomplete or indecipherable data.

The Uncomputer Age

It's been thirty years since I first started practicing medicine, and the advances in technology often baffle me. I have to study and work hard to stay on the leading edge of life in the information age. Sometimes I feel like roadkill on the information highway, but computers undoubtedly offer us the best hope of improving the growing communication vacuum between doctors, pharmacists, and patients.

Adverse drug reactions often result from incomplete or indecipherable data.

Computers run our world . . . except in the area of traditional outpatient medicine. We can't imagine booking a flight, having our electricity hooked up, or registering our car without the use of computers. But did you know *almost all communication between all doctors caring for a particular patient is still either handwritten or dictated and then transcribed by a medical transcriptionist?*

Dark Ages? Consider this. When I see a patient who is also seeing a cardiologist, I will usually receive the cardiologist's clinic notes since I am the primary-care physician. But the cardiologist must first dictate notes on the patient's visit and then have them transcribed. Often the specialist will then review his dictation and sign it before sending it on to me. Once I receive these clinic notes, I must have my staff pull the patient's chart and place it on my desk for review. Once I have reviewed the notes, I then place them in the chart.

It is not unusual to get these notes three and four weeks after the cardiologist actually saw my patient. When I see that patient again, he or she invariably asks if I received the notes from the cardiologist. Sometimes the notes are in the patient's chart and sometimes they're not. If they're not, I am left to ask the patient what the cardiologist told him. You can imagine, I get some very interesting stories and comments!

When patients are primarily seeing specialists within a multispecialty clinic, the various specialists treating the patient are able to share the same medical record. But many specialists either practice alone or with physicians in their same specialty. In any event, specialists tend to make referrals (usually to other specialists) because of their limited general medical expertise and interest. (This is why they became specialists in the first place; they wanted to focus on only the areas of their specialties.)

For example, if you are seeing your cardiologist and you complain of having bright-red rectal bleeding, he will invariably send you to a gastroenterologist. If you are complaining of a painful swollen knee, you will be sent to the orthopedic surgeon or rheumatologist. Needless to say, all of these physicians need your medical history and will most likely add medications to your medical regimen. Is your medical record readily available?

Every physician attempts to obtain a medical history and tries to document which drugs a patient is taking or may be allergic to. But this means we must rely on the patient's memory to retrieve, in some cases, extremely complicated medical problems in conjunction with multiple medications he or she may be taking. This is not an easy task, especially with our elderly population.

I always review the medication my patients are presently taking. Invariably, most of the time they don't know the names of all the drugs they are taking. If they know the names, they can rarely recall the doses. Usually I must look back at my earlier notes and flow sheet, hoping their files have additional notes that I might have received from specialists they are seeing. Some physicians don't send out notes at all or are very slow when they do.

It's not unusual for a patient to tell me that the cardiologist switched his medication but he can't remember its name. He then quickly informs me that it is the blue capsule with the white stripe around the middle. Pausing for a moment, he'll then say that the allergist also just switched him to a pink tablet that replaced the yellow one. When I ask if I can look at the medication, he'll slowly shake his head, realizing he left it all at home. And this describes a good visit.

I always keep an updated record of every medication my patients are taking and the dose of each particular medication. In fact, my nurses go over this in detail with them before each clinic visit. We put all of this information on a flow sheet in the front of the medical chart. Still, some of my patients have seen three or four different specialists since the last visit I had with them. I may have reports from a couple of the specialists, but rarely do I know exactly everything that has transpired with my patient.

Jim's Story

Jim was a local stockbroker with a driven personality and, as a result, he was a self-made success—financial success, that is. For all he accomplished in his career, he managed to neglect his personal care. The only exercise the stockbroker got was stepping into a golf cart and lifting a can of soda or beer between his swings. He had gained a significant amount of weight during his thirties and eventually ended up with fairly high blood pressure.

Now, at age sixty-seven, Jim was seeing his share of doctors.

Initially, his doctor placed him on a calcium channel blocker called Norvasc. This helped, but did not control, his blood pressure. Therefore, he added Lotensin, an ACE inhibitor. These medications did a fair job of controlling his blood pressure for several years, but Jim slowly developed increasing levels of cholesterol and triglycerides—while his good cholesterol (HDL cholesterol) dropped, his bad cholesterol (LDL cholesterol) increased. He also began to experience chest pains while walking up stairs or small inclines.

Jim's primary-care physician, who had placed him on Celebrex for his arthritis, referred him to a local cardiologist, who performed an exercise stress test. The results looked good, but during the stress test Jim's blood pressure went up higher than the cardiologist liked. He added a beta-blocker called Tenormin to his regimen, and because of his high cholesterol and triglycerides, he also prescribed Lipitor.

Jim did well for the next couple of years, but during his annual checkup his chemistry profile revealed elevated blood sugar. He was definitely diabetic, so his primary-care physician referred him to the endocrinologist, who gave brief instructions in diet and exercise while writing out scripts for Glucophage and Glucotrol. Jim did eventually see the diabetic nurse and dietician but only halfheartedly followed their recommendations before giving up completely. He did a poor job of controlling his diabetes, and his endocrinologist gave him repeated warnings about trying to watch his diet better.

Over time Jim's weight had strained his joints, and soon he was having terrible pain in both knees and his left hip. Jim consulted an orthopedic surgeon, who said that he would need a joint replacement in his right knee. The left knee and left hip would soon follow. Because Jim was relatively young, the orthopedic surgeon decided simply to continue him on Celebrex, which is a nonsteroidal anti-inflammatory, hoping to delay surgery.

Not only was Jim's health failing, but his business was as well. Caught in a major crisis following a sharp drop in the stock market, he began experiencing anxiety attacks from time to time. Soon the stockbroker's anxiety turned to depression, so he made an appointment with a psychiatrist. After listening intently, the psychiatrist started Jim on Prozac for the depression and Klonopin (a tranquilizer) for his anxiety.

Jim no longer saw his family doctor, primarily because he was seeing so many specialists. He was having difficulty remembering the medications he was on, and most of his doctors were not aware of all of them either. At one point his endocrinologist sat down with him to figure out all the drugs he was taking, but Jim couldn't recall all their names. His head hurt just trying to think about it.

He explained that he took the slightly yellow pill twice a day, and he thought that was for his arthritis; and he took three different medications for his blood pressure. He used to take a blue capsule, but the last time he saw the cardiologist he had switched from that medication to some samples that came in a red box. The psychiatrist had increased his Prozac to 40 mg each day (he remembered that name) and added a new pill he thought was called Buspar. He told the endocrinologist he had just seen the ophthalmologist, who had noted developing diabetic retinopathy and glaucoma. "Oh, yes," Jim explained, "she started me on some eyedrops—but shoot, I can't remember the name." The endocrinologist was frustrated by this time and simply asked Jim to bring in all of his medications the next time he made an appointment.

Two weeks later Jim began to develop a harsh cough. He had been working long hours while trying to keep his business on track. After three days of fighting a sore throat and cough, he developed a fever. Feeling desperate, he decided to stop by the urgent-care center late at night on his way home. While filling out the paperwork, he felt like a toasted marshmallow and could remember only three of the drugs he was taking. He knew he had reacted to an antibiotic before but just couldn't remember which one it was. The physician's assistant in urgent care believed he had developed bronchitis and prescribed Cipro. She figured this was a safe choice since Jim's allergic reaction had probably happened years before this new drug had been released.

Jim recovered from the bronchitis without incident but continued to ignore all of his physicians' advice until two weeks before his sixty-third birthday, when he developed severe, crushing substernal chest pressure that radiated down his left arm. His family rushed him to the emergency room where the doctor informed Jim that he was having a heart attack.

The cardiologist performed an emergency cardiac catheterization and found that Jim had significant narrowing of all his arteries. The main artery going down the front of his heart was completely closed off, so they performed an emergency angioplasty and inserted a device called a stent to hold the artery open. Jim survived the heart attack and the angioplasty and went home a week later.

Jim never returned to work and remains in extremely poor health. Because of his deteriorated condition, he has never been able to have his joints replaced, so he lives in significant pain. He continues to see all of his specialists but has recently been seeing a neurologist too, because he has been having small transient strokes. The neurologist suggested Coumadin because his patient had now developed atrial fibrillation (irregular heartbeats).

The neurologist has since sent Jim back to his cardiologist to deal with the rhythm problem of his heart. But in order to see the cardiologist, Jim had to cancel his appointment with the urologist, which he had scheduled because of erectile dysfunction. Instead, he decided to call an 800 number he had been carrying around in his billfold for the past six months to see if the phone doctor would prescribe Viagra. The phone doctor ordered the Viagra for Jim, feeling it would be safe since Jim was not taking any nitroglycerin medication. The cardiologist then confirmed that he had atrial fibrillation and placed him on Betapace and took him off the Tenormin. He also agreed with the neurologist that he should continue with the Coumadin and even added Plavix.

Doesn't all this sound absurd? Believe it; I've heard many more like it.

Jim came to see me, feeling he needed a primary-care physician who might possibly eliminate some of his medications and just help him to keep track of everything. He was right. Jim was taking Betapace, Plavix, Coumadin, Viagra, Timoptic eyedrops, Norvasc, Lotensin, Prozac, Buspar, Klonopin, Lipitor, Glucophage, Glucotrol, Celebrex, and Tylenol with codeine. By my calculations, Jim had been seeing seven different physicians during the past year, and they were all individually prescribing him medications.

Jim's situation was a complicated and serious one that would take hard work to unravel. After mixing and matching medications while neglecting his health and his medical history for so long, he was extremely fortunate not to have encountered a drug interaction. His story will conclude in the next chapter.

Getting comprehensive medical care in our world today is not an easy task and often requires many different physicians. Physicians are disease- and drug-oriented. It is nearly impossible for a patient to consult a physician and leave his office without receiving at least one prescription. After all, this is what we doctors do best.

Physicians love to add drugs but really hate to take them away. Remember this general rule: the more physicians involved, the more drugs you will be taking. As you begin to develop health problems, you can anticipate that your health-care providers will prescribe exponential amounts of medication. Never forget: the more drugs you are taking, the greater risk you will have for a severe adverse drug reaction.

CHAPTER TEN

Polypharmacy

TAKE A MOMENT TO BE REALLY HONEST WITH YOURSELF. WHAT is your personal attitude toward medication? Better yet, set the book down and count the number of drugs in your purse, car, drawers, refrigerator, kitchen cupboards, bathroom cabinets, and bedroom closets (how about your desk at the office?). Write the number up in the corner of this page. Do you automatically think about finding relief as soon as you feel pain or discomfort? Your drug inventory may prove shocking.

The tremendous marketing by the pharmaceutical companies, and their support in the health-care system and media, has conditioned most of us to go directly to the cabinet for Tylenol, Motrin, or aspirin when we get a headache. With an upset stomach, we reach for Tagamet, Axid, or Pepcid. And when flu season rolls around we stock up on cough syrups, decongestants, or sinus-flu medications.

The pharmaceutical industry has provided us with an abundance of effective medications, and the use of these drugs saves and significantly changes many lives. In tandem with physicians who are willing to readily prescribe drugs to their patients, however, we have developed an exaggerated dependence on the use of medications. Pharmaceuticals are a booming industry, and our reliance on their medications guarantees repeat business—it's the name of the game.

An Overmedicated Nation

The United States and many modernized nations have made the decision to relieve illness and the complications of chronic degenerative disease processes largely with the use of pharmaceutical drugs. In response to the escalating costs of pharmaceutical drugs, our government, physicians, and insurance companies have determined that the best way to bring down the cost of medicine is to medicate patients earlier in the disease process. We find this to be overwhelmingly true in cases of hypertension, heart disease, arthritis, diabetes, Alzheimer's dementia, Parkinson's disease, and so on.

We have developed an exaggerated dependence on the use of medications.

Physicians have come to believe that medication can alter the long-term complications of many of these diseases, and they hope even to slow down the disease process. This mind-set, which pharmaceutical companies readily encourage, is something medical practitioners wholeheartedly accept as they rely on present medications while waiting for future advances in pharmaceutical discoveries.

We've come to believe that the benefits of medication far outweigh the risks in patients—even for those taking lifelong drugs that treat various chronic degenerative diseases. Consider the amount of medication physicians currently prescribe for high blood pressure, heart disease, diabetes, elevated cholesterol, and arthritis alone. Then add prescriptions for depression, weight loss, sleep, anxiety, infections, asthma, allergies, and cold/pain remedies, and you catch a glimpse of our society's enormous dependence on medication. This approach has been at the forefront of medicine for the past thirty to forty years.

Pharmaceutical companies have been delighted with this approach and offer undying support with a continual barrage of new drugs. In 1960, only 650 medications were available in the U.S. Now we boast more than 8,000.[1] Physicians can prescribe drugs for almost any condition, and if we don't presently have an applicable one, we will soon.

Do you ever wonder at the new diseases created to sell more medication? For example, Paxil and Zoloft, which were released on the market to treat depression, have now been approved to treat "social anxiety disorder." Patients with "social anxiety disorder" have difficulty being around other people in a social situation. Both Zoloft and Paxil are now approved for this use by the FDA. The pharmaceutical reps are now encouraging doctors to look for and make this diagnosis so we can prescribe their company's drug. Patients have been shown to have improvement with this problem using this medication. This is a great example of how a drug is targeted to treat a disease or disorder that was not previously recognized—or at least I had never considered treating it with a medication.

> In 1960, only 650 medications were available in the U.S. Now we boast more than 8,000.

Pharmaceutical companies have certainly been effective in promoting the idea that menopause is a disease requiring a lifetime of hormonal replacement. Although this attitude is changing, Premarin is the most prescribed medication in the world today. I find this statistic staggering, especially with the realization that Premarin is only prescribed for women who have entered menopause. Recent studies are now encouraging women to consider getting off of their hormone replacement therapy if it is being used primarily for the prevention of degenerative diseases, and not for menopausal symptoms.[2]

The amount of prescription meds, over-the-counter drugs, and herbal therapies we consume in our modern-day world is overwhelming. When was the last time you went to the pharmacy to get a prescription filled? *Did you even consider a treatment other than medication?* Did you have the doctor simply call in the script to the pharmacy so you would not have to wait? Did the pharmacist update your record as to other medications you may be taking or those to which you may have reacted recently? Did he personally instruct you about the precautions you should take when using this new medication? Did you receive an information sheet? Did you take time to read it?

Though there's definitely a place for medications in all of our lives, my hope is that we will begin to use them less frequently and more judiciously to decrease potential harmful effects. The goal is to know the inherent risks involved and to make fully informed choices.

In order to do so efficiently, we must centralize our medical care and health records with the help of a primary-care physician, as I described in the previous chapter. But there's another important step. Let us now look at the next vital link involved in the use of prescription medication—the pharmacy.

The Pharmacy Connection

Pharmacists are a critical link in the chain of protection against an adverse drug reaction. Being trained in the actions, interactions, and safety of medications, they are the final safety net for prescription drugs. Pharmacists not only have the training but the tools to protect you.

One of the most important roles a pharmacist has is to inform the doctor that he has requested a medication to which the patient is allergic. Did you know most pharmacies keep an updated record of any drugs you have reacted to when they have received the necessary information? The pharmacist also maintains a list of all the medications you are already taking. Built into most pharmacy computers today is software that detects possible drug interactions so that in the event a physician prescribes two drugs that are known to potentially interact in a harmful way, a warning comes up on the screen.

Computers are invaluable in protecting us against known serious drug interactions—but only to the extent that the pharmacist can enter complete and correct data. When he has sufficient information, he can consult the prescribing physician to discuss any potential problems with the drug he or she just prescribed. This is a critical step in your protection. The prescribing physician may be completely unaware of a potential interaction with another medication a different physician prescribed. Needless to say, pharmacists don't simply count pills and type up the directions.

Pharmacists have also become the *main source* of information for patients regarding side effects and potential dangers of medications. Most pharmacies now give their customers an information sheet listing all the basic information of each drug the first time they fill the prescription (most pharmacies do not provide the information with refills). Table 1 illustrates an example of an information sheet a pharmacist provided for a quinolone antibiotic.

Table 1

Directions for a Fluroquinolone Antibiotic

USES:
This medication is a quinolone antibiotic used to treat certain types of infections (e.g., respiratory tract infections, sinus infections, and urinary tract infections).

HOW TO USE:
Take this medication by mouth, generally once daily, as directed by your doctor. Drink plenty of fluids while using this drug, unless instructed otherwise. The length of treatment depends on your condition and response to therapy. Take this medication exactly as prescribed. Do not exceed the recommended dose of this medication. Antibiotics work best when the amount of medicine in your body is kept at a constant level. This is done by taking the medication at evenly spaced intervals (e.g., every 24 hours). Continue to take this medication until the full-prescribed amount is finished, even if symptoms disappear after a few days. Stopping the medicine too early may allow bacteria to continue to grow resulting in a relapse of the infection. Avoid taking didanosine, sucralfate, aluminum/magnesium-containing antacids, iron or zinc preparations, or vitamin/mineral products within 4 hours of taking this medicine. These products may bind with this medicine and interfere with its absorption. Consult your pharmacist for more information.

SIDE EFFECTS:
Nausea, stomach pain, diarrhea, mild dizziness or headache may occur. If any of these effects persist or worsen, notify your doctor promptly. Tell your doctor immediately if you have any of these unlikely but serious side effects: white patches in the mouth, unusual vaginal itching or discharge. Tell your doctor immediately if you have any of these very unlikely but serious side effects: unusually fast/slow/irregular pulse, chest pain, seizure, mental/mood changes, muscle/tendon pain or swelling, fainting. Allergic reactions to this drug are unlikely, but seek immediate medical attention if they occur. Symptoms of an allergic reaction include: rash, itching, swelling, dizziness, trouble breathing. If you notice other effects not listed above, contact your doctor or pharmacist.

PRECAUTIONS:
Tell your doctor your medical history, including: allergies (especially to quinolone antibiotics such as ciprofloxacin), kidney disease, diabetes, seizures, tendon problems (e.g., tendonitis, bursitis), heart problems (e.g., QTc interval proloration, bradycardia, arrythmia, myocardial

Table 1, continued

infaction), brain disorders (e.g., cerebral atherosclerosis, tumors or increased intracranial pressure), low blood potassium (hypokalemia). This drug may make you dizzy. Use caution engaging in activities requiring alertness such as driving or using machinery. Limit alcohol intake because it can intensify the dizziness effect of this medication. Use of this medication for prolonged or repeated periods may result in a secondary infection (e.g., oral, bladder or vaginal yeast infection). Patients with diabetes may experience changes in blood sugar due to infection or use of this medication. Monitor your blood glucose levels frequently while using this medication and notify your doctor promptly if you experience symptoms of high or low blood sugar. Symptoms of high blood sugar include increased thirst and urination. Symptoms of low blood sugar include dizziness, sweating, hunger and fast pulse. Though gatifloxacin has not been shown to make skin sensitive to the sun, other drugs very similar to this one have. Therefore, avoid excessive sunlight and sun lamps. Consult your doctor or pharmacist for more information. This medication should be used with caution in children less than 18 years of age. This medication may cause joint or bone problems in young children. This medication should be used only when clearly needed during pregnancy. Discuss the risks and benefits with your doctor. It is not known whether this drug passes into breast milk. Consult your doctor before breast-feeding.

DRUG INTERACTIONS:
Tell your doctor of all prescription and nonprescription medication you may use, especially of: drugs for diabetes (e.g., glyburide, insulin), NSAIDs (e.g., ibuprofen, naproxen), drugs that decrease potassium levels such as certain "water pills" (e.g., furosemide, hydrochlorothiazide), drugs for irregular heartbeat (e.g., quinidine, procianamide, disopyramide, amiodarone, sotalol), tricyclic antidepressants (e.g., amitriptyline, nortriptyline), phenothiazine drugs (e.g., chlorpromazine, prochlorperazine, perphenazine), didanosine, sucralfate, digoxin, probenecid, warfarin,magnesium/aluminum-containing antacids, iron preparations, zinc supplements, vitamin/mineral supplements, cisapride, erythromycin, astemizole, terfenadine. Also report use of drugs that may affect the heart (prolong the QTc interval) such as: pentamidine, pimozide, halofantrine, bepridil. Do not start or stop any medicine without doctor or pharmacist approval.

MISSED DOSE:
If you miss a dose, use it as soon as you remember. If it is near the time of the next dose, skip the missed dose and resume your usual dosing schedule. Do not double the dose to catch up.

Although these information sheets are insightful, they by no means tell the whole story. They primarily point out the most *common* or the most *serious* potential side effects of each drug. And many times the sheet describes the *symptoms* of a potential side effect rather than the specific reaction itself. For example, the information sheet will explain that your skin may turn yellow or your stools might become pale, or you may experience abdominal pain. In this case, the underlying reaction is really potential liver damage; these are merely descriptions of the symptoms that you might notice.

With the many resources available in books and the Internet, we have no shortage of information available for the drugs we are taking. *But understanding and effectively using the information can prove to be a challenge indeed.* After reading the information in Table 1, you probably found that most of this information is not only difficult for the average person to understand; it is like a foreign language. At the end of this book you will find a list of resources available to the public to learn more about the particular drugs you are taking.

Although the information sheets are insightful, they by no means tell the whole story.

Americans are independent and capitalistic. We appreciate our freedom in researching and managing the details of our family's health as well as budgeting our time, money, and resources. In our usual manner of being resourceful, we pick and choose our medications, doctors, and pharmacies with the same mentality we use when shopping for groceries or hiring a plumber. Customer loyalty is a thing of the past. We will shop where the best quality is offered for the lowest price. Comparative shopping is the best way to go when buying furniture or shoes, but when purchasing prescription drugs, we must decide what is most cost-effective in light of our fullest protection.

Missing the Safety Net: Why Pharmacies Are Ineffective in Protecting You

As I've mentioned, pharmacies are the final safety net in discovering and preventing adverse drug reactions. But with the death toll so high, we must ask, what has gone wrong? Why aren't pharmacists stopping more adverse reactions before they start?

In a very real sense doctors and pharmacists hold up one side of the safety net and patients hold the other. Teamwork is imperative here. The physician, pharmacist, and patient must all work together to prevent potential injuries and deaths. In order for dangerous drug interactions to be detected, several troublesome factors must be overcome. *Polypharmacy* is one of them.

Medical literature uses the term *polypharmacy* when referring to patients who are taking several different medications. But after meeting patients like Jim in Chapter 9, I have expanded the term also to include the use of *many different pharmacies*. This term adequately describes patients who typically see several different physicians, who in turn prescribe a variety of drugs that any number of different pharmacies fill.

Jim offers a case in point.

Jim's Story, Continued

Prior to his visit with me, Jim didn't know the benefits of utilizing the centralized care of a family physician. Even though he initially had a primary-care physician, once he became ill and had began seeing several different specialists, he decided he did not need to see his primary-care doctor anymore. For years he bounced from one specialist to another without following through on most of his doctors' recommendations. Not only had he received mixed messages from time to time, his approach to health care afforded little accountability or follow-up. As Paul Harvey would say, "Now, for the rest of the story."

Comparative shopping is the best way to go when buying furniture or shoes, but when purchasing prescription drugs, we must decide what is most cost-effective in light of our fullest protection.

Jim was not an unusual patient and like many others who walk into my office, he was in serious trouble. Not only was he seeing many specialists, further problems with his medical care came to light when I discovered how he went about having prescriptions filled.

My new patient was having his Plavix, Prozac, Betapace, Norvasc,

Buspar, Lipitor, and Celebrex prescriptions filled through a mail-in pharmacy that his insurance carrier supported. By doing so, he was able to get a ninety-day supply of each medication for a reasonable cost, especially compared to what it would cost him at a local pharmacy. But others of his drugs—Coumadin, Glucophage, Glucotrol, Tylenol with codeine, and Lotensin—cost less money at a local pharmacy. Several of these drugs were generic, and because Jim needed to keep changing his dose of the Coumadin, it was more convenient to use the local pharmacy.

Jim was getting his Timoptic eyedrops from the pharmacy located in his ophthalmolgist's clinic, and his phone doctor prescribed Viagra through a different mail-in pharmacy from his regular one. Finally, when Jim had gone to the urgent-care clinic during his bout with bronchitis, he had his prescription for Cipro filled in a twenty-four-hour pharmacy located on the other side of town because it was on his way home. According to my calculations, he had been using five different pharmacies to obtain his medications within the previous six months. It was time for a change.

First, I requested that Jim have all of his specialists send me their office notes so I could consolidate his medical record. After corresponding with some of them, I was able to assume the primary management of his care and refer him back to them only when necessary.

Next, we went to work on his prescription use. Jim desired to make some significant lifestyle changes in the hopes that he could reduce use of some of his medications. In addition to a simple but healthy diet, I started Jim on glucosamine sulfate and a potent nutritional supplement used for degenerative arthritis. After four months he discontinued the Tylenol with codeine on his own and used Celebrex only occasionally for arthritis pain.

Within a few months, his diabetes came under excellent control and he was able to discontinue Glucotrol. As a result of a balanced diet and stable blood sugar levels, Jim began feeling much better and less depressed. I was then able to suggest that he discontinue both his Buspar and Prozac. His cardiologist also switched him from Plavix to a baby aspirin each day.

Jim is slowly improving and will hopefully be able to ease off more of his medication over time. For now, he is purchasing all of his meds through the same pharmacy, and he has a list of all his medications in his billfold. He told me during the last visit that he hasn't felt this good in years.

Jim's story sounds somewhat extreme, but isn't it true that most of us consider shopping and comparing costs for our prescriptions an economical and wise use of our hard-earned money? How many patients actually use a single pharmacy? Studies indicate that more than 40 percent of Americans receive care from more than one physician, and 33 percent of patients use more than one pharmacy to get their medications filled.[3]

Using more than one pharmacy is definitely more common in patients who are taking several different drugs. But you must be aware that physicians do not always keep track of where patients have their scripts filled. Pharmacies generally do not share information. And when the pharmacy does not have a list of all the drugs you are taking, its software cannot possibly evaluate potential drug interactions.

Miscommunication

Do you remember the game "Telephone" that we played as kids when trapped inside on a rainy day? We'd sit in a circle and one person would start by saying something silly like, "I love to ride my bicycle in the rain." Then each child would whisper what he heard to the person sitting next to him. "I ride my bicycle for a tan." "I sold my bike to Dan."

The telephone game teaches many children a life lesson on how the retelling easily loses or scrambles details. You may chuckle as you remember sitting next to that boy with cooties who got your message all mixed up or other times in a real-life situation when gossip got out of hand. But nowhere is it more imperative for people to clearly communicate detailed facts than in the medical field. The physician must correctly communicate messages to the pharmacist, and then to the patient. What is the margin of error? How many distractions and interruptions possibly skew the original message about prescription medications each day?

Physician to Pharmacy

Have you ever tried to read the prescription (the scribbled print on the little white piece of paper) that your doctor hands you? I know my handwriting is difficult to read. I have had patients ask me if physicians still write prescriptions in Latin. I've even had patients become concerned enough to ask me how a pharmacist actually interprets what I have just written. I typically become concerned after these friendly reminders, becoming more diligent with neatness for a while. But then the busier I get, the poorer my handwriting becomes again.

Pharmacists have not yet been required to take a special course in hieroglyphics, but it's obviously very important for them to be able to read what we doctors have written on the prescription. A misinterpretation of the script can and does cause serious adverse drug reactions. Mistakes happen.

You may feel relieved to know that your particular doctor *calls* your prescriptions in directly to the pharmacist. Unfortunately this, too, has its drawbacks. In the first place, it is rare to actually speak to a pharmacist anymore. They are too busy filling other scripts. A pharmacy tech often takes the information over the phone from the doctor or the doctor's nurse.

> Roughly one-quarter of all reported drug errors involve drug name mix-ups.

Most often when I call in a prescription, I talk to a machine that records the information. This procedure may not seem alarming at first, because we are so reliant on automated technical devices like answering machines and voice mail. But Bruce Lambert, Ph.D., an associate professor of pharmacy administration at the University of Illinois, reported that roughly one-quarter of all reported drug errors involve *drug name mix-ups.*[4]

For instance, a doctor may be calling in medication formerly called Losec, which at one time pharmacists commonly mistook for Lasix. Its manufacturer eventually changed the name to Prilosec because of the mistakes. Now there are reports that pharmacists have mistakenly given

Prilosec for Prozac, an antidepressant drug. Other common mix-ups include

- Aminophylline for Amitriptyline
- Digoxin for digitoxin
- Nicoderm for Nitroderm
- Haldol for Halcion
- Urax for Eurax
- Xanax for Zantac[5]

You can see how easy it would be to confuse some of these names! According to the FDA, medication mix-ups cause roughly one death per day.[6] Many of these errors lead to serious adverse drug reactions that lead even to hospitalization. One patient noted that the pharmacist gave him a prescription for Viagra when the doctor had ordered Allegra (an antihistamine). The patient became concerned when his "antihistamine" cost so much more than he expected.

Pharmacist to Patient

The physician/pharmacy/patient team connection often suffers a breakdown in communicating vital information between physician and pharmacist, but errors are also commonplace between pharmacy and patient. Pharmacists are also extremely busy, and when they do take time to talk to the patient individually they are often rushed, leaving patients more confused than ever. Overworked pharmacists may also miss critical drug interactions, which may lead to serious adverse drug reactions.

> According to the FDA, medication mix-ups cause roughly one death per day.

A study done in cooperation with the Georgetown University School of Medicine looked at how efficient pharmacies were in warning patients about possible dangerous drug interactions. Seven physician-pharmacologists wrote prescriptions for three different drug combinations known to cause potentially serious reactions when taken together. Undercover investigators presented these scripts, at the same time, to 245 different pharmacies to be filled.

More than half of the pharmacies failed to warn the consumers against the dangers of mixing these drugs. A pharmacist was considered to have given a warning if he counseled the patient, offered to call the doctor, or refused to fill the prescriptions. Here are some of the findings of this survey:

- Approximately one-third of the pharmacists did not alert consumers to the potentially severe interaction between Hismanal, a common antihistamine, and Nizoral, an often-prescribed antifungal drug. The Hismanal-Nizoral mix can cause cardiac arrest and death. This is the same reaction that can occur between Seldane and Nizoral or Erythromycin. Hismanal and Seldane have since been taken off the market.
- Only four out of seventeen pharmacies warned of acute interaction between oral contraceptives and Rimactane, an antibiotic used to treat tuberculosis, which diminishes the effect of birth-control drugs and can render them ineffective.
- Fewer than half the pharmacies surveyed included the information sheets, which list the warnings and possible interactions of the medications, with the prescriptions.
- Independent pharmacies and pharmacies located in low- to lower-middle-income neighborhoods accounted for the largest number of pharmacies that failed to warn the consumer about the potential dangers of these drug combinations.[7]

This study involved drugs that could cause potentially serious problems when taken at the same time. Imagine the results if a study were done where a drugstore filled these scripts two months apart or even six months apart. The implications of this study suggest that the majority of pharmacies are not focused on detecting drug interactions.

Another margin of error comes as a result of pharmacists' wrongly dispensing drugs. Just as drugs have similar-sounding names, many drugs have similar packaging. A number of drug errors reported to the FDA occurred when the pharmacist pulled the wrong drug off the shelf. It makes good sense for patients always to check out the prescriptions they receive from the pharmacy, making sure they have the correct names, dosages, and directions the physician prescribed. If this is a refill of a medication you have already been taking, compare the shape, color, and size of the pills. If there is a difference, question the pharmacist about why it is different. Blind faith is never sufficient. If you have any hesitation, if an explanation wasn't clear, no matter how long the line behind you—ask. If you have a nagging question lingering in your mind, ask, always ask—a life may depend on it.

> If you have a nagging question lingering in your mind, ask, always ask—a life may depend on it.

Alfred's Story

I look forward to visiting with pharmaceutical reps when they come by my office. Mine is a much different attitude than most physicians have; they often complain about how much time the reps consume and how many there are now. Even though I, too, wish there were not so many of them, I allow two of them a day to share their products with me in my office, and once a week I allow a rep to bring my staff lunch. This provides him more time to inform me about a company's latest developments.

During one of these lunches, I shared with a pharmaceutical rep about this book I am writing on adverse drug reactions. He became quite interested, and we visited at some length about what I had been learning and writing. He wrapped up our brief visit by telling me a humorous story about his grandfather, Alfred, in Nebraska.

Alfred's health had been declining for several years, and his family finally placed him in a nursing home at the age of eighty-nine. Due to his plethora of ailments, Alfred was taking approximately twelve different medications. As time passed the elderly grandpa became so weak he couldn't eat food or swallow his medication.

Knowing that his death was near, his physician chose the most merciful treatment—discontinuing all medication while offering daily supportive care. The doctor then called the whole family. His patient was dying, he said, and if they wanted to see him they needed to come immediately.

The family rushed to Alfred's side and waited for him to die. "Grandpa was as frail as an autumn leaf. His respirations were so shallow that the doctor told us it would be only a matter of a day or two before he would pass away," said the pharmaceutical rep. "So the whole family waited . . . and waited, and waited. But Grandpa didn't die. In fact, he started to become more alert and began responding to the family. It wasn't long before he was asking for water and then food."

The rep concluded, "Grandpa Alfred just celebrated his ninety-third birthday and is now actually healthier than he's been in years!" The elderly man has never taken any more medication and, in retrospect, the family has no doubt that the mix of all the different medications was responsible for Alfred's decline and near-death.

The Blame Game: A Summary

If you develop an adverse drug reaction, whose fault is it anyway? There is always plenty of blame to go around. When a drug has the desired result, everyone is happy. But when a drug has an unwanted result, and a patient is injured or dies, everyone points his finger at someone else as having the primary fault. I call this the Blame Game.

In Part II of this book we've discovered the different links in a chain of events directly affecting the safety of every single medication ever prescribed. Here I'll encapsulate in brief review the different reasons a patient can experience an adverse drug reaction.

Pharmaceutical Companies and the FDA

Since Congress passed the PDUFA legislation in 1992, the FDA no longer plays an adversarial role against the pharmaceutical companies.

Instead, the legislation made them partners. "User fees" make up approximately 50 percent of the FDA's budget and have allowed pharmaceutical companies to place certain demands on the FDA. Congress has placed the FDA under tough production guidelines, so that it must work together with the pharmaceutical industry to approve as many drugs as possible.

Pharmaceutical companies have a role in this whole process that everyone can understand: they are interested in getting safe and effective drugs approved by the FDA as quickly as possible. Their goals and desires are easy to predict. The difference in the last few years is the fact that the FDA is actually listening and catering to the industry's desires. The FDA, in essence, is facilitating the entire new drug-approval process. And why shouldn't it? After all, pharmaceutical companies are footing the bill. Drug companies are accountable to their stockholders and need to create a profit. Do they want safe and effective drugs? Of course they do. The more effective and safe the drug, the better it is for the pharmaceutical company and the stockholders. Everybody wants a winner.

Any serious adverse drug reaction the Postmarketing Surveillance Department of the FDA identifies must be referred to the same FDA advisory committee that originally approved the drug. It is very difficult for that committee to admit it may have made a mistake in originally approving the drug. It is in no way an impartial jury. The FDA does not want to see these drugs withdrawn from the market.

If a drug *has* to be withdrawn, the FDA has the perfect out: it can blame the doctors. We are talking *prescription* medications, after all. The FDA is placing these drugs in the physicians' care. It is the doctors' responsibility to evaluate the clinical situation and prescribe medications properly.

Most serious adverse reactions (the ones that are known) have been spelled out in the drug information packet every physician should read and understand. Ultimately, this takes the FDA and pharmaceutical companies off the hook. The pharmaceutical companies did their job by properly performing the requirements necessary to have the FDA approve their new drug application. The FDA has done its job by properly informing physicians of potential problems with each new drug it approved.

When problems arise after a drug has been released, the FDA properly informs health-care providers of any and all label warnings via the MedWatch program. If there are serious complications, the pharmaceutical company also contacts the physician via a "Dear Doctor" letter.

The Physician

What is the physician's part in the blame game? I am going to answer this question from my thirty years of clinical experience; because I'm not aware of any studies that address this question. I am certain, however, that I can come close in eliciting the top physician responses.

The number-one response would be to blame the inherent risk of medication. That is right: we blame the medications themselves. Every day of our careers we must weigh the risk of prescribing a particular medication against the potential benefits of the medication. You can't practice medicine very long without encountering a poor result due to an adverse drug reaction.

For example, we use Coumadin quite frequently in patients who have atrial fibrillation (an irregular heart rhythm in which the upper and lower chambers of the heart are not beating in coordination) to decrease their risk of having a stroke. Yet there is a definite increased risk of spontaneous bleeding. As a result, physicians monitor protimes frequently in order to determine how "thin" the patient's blood has become because of the effects of the Coumadin. The chance of a serious adverse drug reaction with the use of Coumadin, we believe, simply comes with the territory.

Physicians are usually too busy to sit down and tell every patient about all the potential side effects of the drugs they are prescribing, even if they knew what all of the side effects were. Most doctors believe pharmacists are the ones who should be informing patients all about their drugs. If there is a side effect that catches our patient unaware, we can always blame the pharmacist.

The last person doctors blame is the patient. We figure he didn't listen well enough to the instructions and failed to take the medicine(s) properly. A classic casting of blame is this one: "The patient should have reported her symptoms earlier if she was having problems."

The Pharmacist

Pharmacists are the only ones in this whole chain of events specifically trained in pharmacology. Their training allows them to recognize and alert the patient and physician to potential problems. They act as the safety net in protecting the physician, who may have ordered a drug to which the patient is known to be allergic, or perhaps ordered a drug in the wrong dose. The pharmacist should be instructing the patient in detail about the potential risks and side effects of the drug. But I am sure they, too, have their own list of people and agencies to blame.

They certainly rely on the FDA to keep them completely informed about any new developments or decisions it has made. The pharmacists supply patients with a computerized sheet on all the do's and don'ts of each medication. Pharmacists can blame the patient if he does not read and follow their instructions. Furthermore, patients often get their medications from several different pharmacies. How can pharmacists be expected to keep track of possible drug interactions?

The Patient

Patients are the most innocent players in this entire chain of events. They trust their doctors, they trust the FDA, they trust their pharmacists, and they even trust pharmaceutical companies. When they suffer from an adverse drug reaction, they usually want to be understanding. If the ADR leaves them with a permanent injury, however, this understanding quickly changes to confusion and then anger.

At first, patients don't quite understand how it could happen. A drug reaction was the last thing they would ever expect. They not only become bitter, but often they will blame everyone involved. Most often neither their doctors nor their pharmacists told them that this particular adverse drug reaction was a possibility.

If the doctors and pharmacies had no idea such a reaction could occur, the patients then feel like guinea pigs. Can you blame them? I surely don't. They were taking the medication with the idea it would help them, not hurt them. Other than medical situations in which the prognosis is serious or terminal, patients are not willing to take any risks with their health or lives.

My patients who actually read the package insert that accompanies some of the sample medications frequently call me up and tell me there is no way they will take a particular medication. Have you ever done that? I suggest that you do. Read one of the package inserts on a drug you are taking or look it up in the *Physicians' Desk Reference* (PDR).

————

I would venture to guess that you had no idea of all the problems your particular medication could possibly cause. Whose fault is it? Do you blame your pharmacist? After all, he did give you an information sheet about your drug when you picked up your medicine. Or did he? Even if he did, that information sheet will not come close to informing you of *all* the possible problems.

Do you blame your doctor? She wrote the prescription. Though she may have warned you of some of the most common side effects of the drug, I know that she didn't tell you all of the possible problems that could result from taking a particular medication—it's not possible. When you develop a serious adverse drug reaction, who is to blame?

You must no longer passively trust a multifaceted chain of events, believing all the while that everything possible is being done to protect you. It is time for a paradigm shift in your health care. Ultimately, you are the only one who can protect yourself from the potential danger of adverse drug reactions. The next section focuses on a new, more informed approach to your self-care. Whether purchasing over-the-counter drugs, herbal therapies, or working to prevent disease through a healthier lifestyle, you can know how to make the safest choice.

PART III

TAKE CHARGE OF YOUR HEALTH

CHAPTER ELEVEN

Over-the-Counter Medications

THE INTRODUCTION OF THIS BOOK OPENED WITH MY THOUGHTS and feelings of despondency as I reflected on the harrowing events of the previous forty-eight hours.

> *A little blonde girl with big round eyes now lay in a children's hospital connected to tubes and IVs, fighting for her life. She had almost died during transport. I glanced at my watch, wondering if Heidi was still alive. Hers was not an anonymous face; Heidi was my patient—the child of a close friend.*

Heidi, the daughter of a local neurologist and my close personal friend, is a beautiful young lady now; however, there were several days when I personally feared for her life. She had developed pneumonia and needed to be admitted to the hospital. I started her on an antibiotic for her pneumonia and treated her fever with acetaminophen. On the second day of her hospital stay she should have been showing improvement, but instead she became more ill with fatigue, nausea, and vomiting.

On the third day blood tests revealed that Heidi's liver enzymes were increasing, which means she was showing evidence that her liver was being damaged, and she was becoming jaundiced. Her condition steadily grew worse with each passing hour. This lovely little girl was fading away right before our eyes. Because her condition was declining rapidly, we discontinued all of her medication in case she was having an adverse drug reaction.

Heidi was so ill at this point that her father and I agreed we needed to transfer her by air ambulance immediately to the University of Minnesota's Children's Hospital, where she could get more specialized care. I was concerned about whether she would survive the flight, and I insisted on attending to her personally en route to Minneapolis.

I traveled with her in case an emergency occurred during the flight. Her respirations were labored, and her color was very poor. The flight took approximately two hours, but it was a lifetime for me. The ground ambulance was waiting for us at the airport in Minneapolis and we rushed my little patient directly to the children's hospital. I was relieved that she was still alive when we finally arrived.

Heidi was admitted directly to the medical intensive care unit, where the pediatrician on call began to evaluate her and quickly called in their pediatric gastroenterologist. He said the initial CT scan showed evidence of severe liver damage. Heidi was experiencing liver failure. The pneumonia was now a minor problem, and they needed to find out what was happening to her liver. The doctor scheduled her for a fine-needle liver biopsy the next day.

I flew back home with the air ambulance crew that night; however, I stayed in close contact with the physicians at the children's hospital. Three days later, they got the liver biopsy back, and indeed she had necrosis of the liver—meaning her liver was basically dying. All the physicians could do was provide support and hope things would turn around.

I was baffled. Heidi's original sickness was now merely a backdrop to the drama of a life-threatening liver condition. With a phone call, I asked the pediatric gastroenterologist what he believed caused her problem in the first place. Without hesitation he replied, "Oh, she's having a severe adverse reaction to acetaminophen."

I paused. I must have sounded dumbfounded when I responded, "To . . . to acetaminophen?"

"Sure," he said, "we see it all the time." The hospital was starting to do liver transplants, and he went on to tell me that most of the patients on the liver-transplant list were children whose livers the drug had destroyed. I had never heard anything like this before in my life. The pediatrician then added, "The combination of Erythromycin, which was needed to treat her mycoplasma pneumonia, and acetaminophen can cause significant stress on anyone's liver, since Erythromycin can accentuate the liver toxicity of the acetaminophen."

I learned many valuable lessons as a young physician, but Heidi's experience left a deep and lasting effect on me. This was the first and most serious drug reaction I had seen. Twenty-five years later, I still get a knot in the pit of my stomach when I think about it.

Thankfully, Heidi fully recovered from this harrowing ordeal. Her father and I continue to be good friends, and I smile every time I see her. To think this reaction was caused by an over-the-counter (OTC) medication still blows my mind. After reading this chapter you, too, will have a different attitude the next time you walk into your local drugstore to buy OTC medication.

Over-the-Counter Drugs: Safe?

Few of us give much thought to drugs like Motrin, Tavist-D, Monistat cream, Aleve, Axid, Pepcid, and hydrocortisone cream. We figure these drugs must be safe—after all, they are over-the-counter. If they were dangerous, the FDA would never allow them to be sold without a prescription, right? Not exactly. Read on.

Since the mid-1970s, the FDA has approved seventy-nine prescription medications to be switched to nonprescription (over-the-counter) status. Thirty-six of these switches occurred in the 1990s alone.[1] As the number of OTC drugs increases, individuals face greater risk as "self-care" patients. When it comes to over-the-counter drugs, this means you are basically on your own.

As never before, you must rely more and more on your own decisions about self-care. Sure, a patient information packet accompanies most OTC drugs, but the risk to you does not change. Did you know that over-the-counter medication causes an estimated sixteen thousand deaths per year?[2]

Did you know that over-the-counter medication causes an estimated sixteen thousand deaths per year?

How many consumers realize that almost all OTC medications were at one time prescription medications? In fact, these drugs are still very similar to many of the medications we physicians are prescribing today. Don't ever think that because they are now available to purchase from your local drugstore they are completely safe. As I learned with little Heidi, we must have the same respect for over-the-counter drugs as we do prescription drugs.

Hazards of Over-the-Counter Meds

- Patients usually do not inform their doctors about OTC drugs they or their children may be taking.
- The overwhelming majority of patients taking OTC drugs do not read or understand the basic side effects and potential adverse drug reactions of the OTC medication they're taking.
- During a mock scenario, only 40 percent of the parents calculated the correct dose of acetaminophen (Tylenol) for their child.
- Overdose and underdosage of OTC medication have led to many ER visits.
- A significant number of caregivers inaccurately administer OTC products to their children.
- Fifty percent of three-year-olds in the United States have received some type of OTC medication during the past year.[3]

Over-the-counter drugs contribute largely to our overmedicated society because we so easily forget to consider them seriously. Conclusive evidence shown in the text box, however, demonstrates how parents have been too relaxed about and trusting of the products on drugstore shelves. We must especially become aware of the potential harm that misuse of these meds can cause children and adolescents. We must aggressively teach our adolescents the inherent danger of all drugs—not just illegal ones. Though adolescents cannot buy cigarettes, they can certainly purchase over-the-counter drugs.

Katie's Story

Katie was a lively teenager who loved music and people. She was involved in both the high school choir and orchestra. Not only was she a good student, she had a caring personality that attracted lots of friends. Wherever Katie was, a group of kids was laughing and having fun.

Ben, one of Katie's classmates, was a shy but attractive boy who had difficulty talking with the girls in his class. He had had a crush on Katie for over a year but was too afraid to ask her out on a real date. His friends would kid him frequently about it, and eventually his fear of rejection faded in comparison to his dread of his friends' teasing. Two months before the big day, Ben finally asked Katie to be his date for the junior-senior prom.

> We must aggressively teach our adolescents the inherent danger of all drugs—not just illegal ones.

Katie graciously accepted his invitation and could hardly wait for the dance. Ben was sweet, and though she wanted to impress him, like most teens Katie was mainly concerned about how she would look that night for all of her friends. Pictures and memories last forever. She had always felt a little self-conscious about being thick around her waist, but now it seemed to be the center of her world. Katie dreamed of how stunning she could be in the gown she and her mom were sewing for the prom.

An advertisement in her favorite teen magazine described an over-the-counter diet pill that seemed to be the perfect solution, since she needed to lose only eight to ten pounds. Katie visited her local drugstore right away and purchased a little box of weight-loss medication from the pharmacy shelf. She couldn't believe how many brands there were to choose from.

Wanting to do everything right, she was careful to take the drug as the box recommended. For the first time in her life, she also decided it was time to get serious about exercising. She wanted this date to be the best night of her life, so she started jogging with some girlfriends. The young teen was surprised at how her appetite lessened and was thrilled to see a noticeable difference around her waist.

Katie's mom admired her daughter's determination to trim down a little. She knew her daughter was a bit concerned about her figure, so she fixed tasty low-cal meals and made certain that Katie and her friends had fresh-cut fruit and veggies available in the refrigerator. She smiled as she watched the girls giggle and talk on the phone for what seemed hours at a time about boys and the prom. How grown-up Katie looked.

About three weeks before the prom, Katie was sitting in choir when she experienced a crushing headache. It started across her forehead and quickly settled down into her neck. Weak and pale, she grabbed the girl next to her, saying she was going to pass out. A minute later, Katie had fallen off her chair, unconscious.

In a frenzy, classmates began crying. The teacher ran to call the ambulance, while some of the students tried to administer CPR. Katie did not respond. The EMT personnel inserted an endotracheal tube so they could ventilate her and continued doing CPR as they rushed the young girl to the local emergency room. There ER physicians continued trying to resuscitate her, but to no avail.

Katie was pronounced dead a mere thirty minutes after her arrival at the emergency room. Her family had not even had time to get to the hospital before she was gone. The whole community shared her family's staggering grief. What had happened?

The ER physicians didn't know. Katie had been unresponsive the entire time of the attempted resuscitation. The ER physicians encouraged Katie's parents to consent to an autopsy. They both agreed.

Five days later, the family doctor called Katie's parents into his office to discuss the results of the autopsy. He informed them that their daughter had suffered a severe hemorrhagic stroke (bleeding into the brain) and never had a chance to survive the assault.

"How does someone as young as Katie have a stroke?" they asked in shock. The doctor said he wasn't sure, but one of Katie's girlfriends had told the EMT personnel that she'd been taking some kind of over-the-counter diet pill. Her mother started sobbing. It seemed like the medical community was coming up with petty excuses for losing her daughter. "What does that have to do with anything?" she cried.

> "How does someone as young as Katie have a stroke?" they asked in shock.

Quietly, but with authority, their doctor explained the drug most likely had *everything* to do with Katie having suffered this type of stroke. He'd done some research after getting the results of the autopsy and had found several cases reporting hemorrhagic stroke in young teenage and adolescent girls taking medications that contained an active ingredient called *phenylpropanolamine*. "In fact," he said, "the FDA is presently considering the removal of all these types of drugs from the market."

Bewildered, Katie's parents tried to process this new information. Their daughter died taking a drug they didn't even know about. Like all parents of teens, they had always been concerned about teens' illicit drug use and had talked openly about the dangers with Katie. The ironic news that their daughter had been snatched away by innocently taking an over-the-counter drug offered no comfort whatsoever. They were outraged. Of all their parental fears, this was one scenario they had never imagined.

Phenylpropanolamine

Phenylpropanolamine (PPA) had already been on the market for two years when the FDA gained needed authority from Congress to regulate the safety of medicines in the year 1938. Therefore, a grandfather clause allowed the drug to stay on the market, even though it was never required to satisfy the testing requirements for new medicines. PPA has since been used in more than four hundred over-the-counter medications during the past seventy-four years. [4] Most of these medications are either cold preparations or over-the-counter weight-loss treatments.

Table 1 lists the most common medications that contained PPA.

Table 1

Over-the-Counter Drugs That Used to Contain PPA

AcuTrim 16-Hour Tablets
AcuTrim Gum
AcuTrim Max Tablets
AcuTrim Maximum Strength Appetite
  Control
Alka-Seltzer Plus Cold Medicine Original
Alka-Seltzer Plus Children's Cold Medicine
  Effervescent
Alka-Seltzer Plus NT
Alka-Seltzer Plus Cold, Cherry
Alka-Seltzer Plus Cold, Orange
Alka-Seltzer Plus Flu Tablets
Alka-Seltzer Plus Sinus
BC Allergy Sinus Cold Powder
BC Sinus Cold Powder
Comtrex Flu Therapy & Fever Relief Day &
  Night
Comtrex Deep Chest
Comtrex Flu Day/Night
Comtrex ND Liquigel
Comtrex 12-Hour Cold Caplets
Comtrex 12-Hour Cold Capsules
CVS Cold & Allergy Elixir DM
CVS Cold & Allergy Tablets Max
CVS Dayhist D, CVS Diet Caplet
CVS Diet Caplet with C
CVS Effervescent Cold Tabs
CVS Triacting Cough
CVS Triacting Expectorant

CVS Triacting Multi
CVS Triacting Multi Cherry
CVS Triacting Sore Throat VS Tussin CF
Dexatrim Caffeine-Free Caplet
Dexatrim Caplet with C Tablet
Dexatrim Gelcaps
Dimetapp Cold & Allergy Chewable
Dimetapp Cold & Cough
Dimetapp Cold & Cough Liqui-Gels
Dimetapp Chew Tabs
Dimetapp DM Cold & Cough Elixir
Dimetapp DM Elixir
Dimetapp Extentabs
Naldecon DX Adult Syrup
Naldecon DX Drops
Naldecon DX Pediatric Drops
Naldecon DX Child Syrup
Parmathene Mega-16
Robitussin Allergy Cough
Robitussin CF
Tavist-D 12-Hour Relief of Sinus & Nasal
  Congestion
Thinz Span Capsules
Triaminic DM Cough Relief
Triaminic Expectorant Chest & Head
  Congestion
Triaminic Syrup Cold & Allergy
Triaminicol C & C

Nearly forty years passed before anyone raised the first concerns of safety. In the 1970s, researchers felt that the increased blood pressure PPA caused could lead to a higher risk of stroke. In 1981, the medical watchdog organization, the Public Citizens' Health Research Group, raised awareness again when it warned against the use of PPA because of concerns about its safety. The FDA even ignored editorials appearing in the *Journal of the American Medical Association* urging health-care providers to avoid products with PPA. Instead, the FDA chose to listen to the pharmaceutical industry, which claimed PPA was safe.[5]

Dr. Raymond Lake, a professor of psychiatry at the University of Kansas, published a review of 142 reported reactions to PPA in

> Could it be possible that a drug that had been on the market for nearly sixty years could be this dangerous?

1989. But follow-up studies reported by Dr. George Blackburn, a nutrition expert at Harvard Medical School, and Dr. John Morgan, a professor of pharmacology at City University of New York, only re-affirmed the safety of PPA, causing a political battle to break out. The Blackburn-Morgan study and follow-up articles all supported the safety of PPA.[6]

The drug had been around so long that everyone quickly dismissed reports of harm. An article that appeared in the *New England Journal of Medicine*, however, started to turn heads when it detailed more than thirty cases of hemorrhagic stroke (bleeding into the brain) that had been reported since 1979 in those having ingested PPA.[7]

Most of the reports involved adolescent girls or young women between the ages of sixteen and twenty-one who were using appetite suppressant drugs containing PPA—just as Katie had.

Intracranial bleeding (hemorrhagic stroke) is a rare occurrence in this age group. Could it be possible that a drug that had been on the market for nearly sixty years could be this dangerous? In addition to these published reports, the FDA admitted that between 1969 and 1991, the agency had received an additional twenty-two reports of hemorrhagic strokes associated with the use of PPA.[8]

Pressure mounted for the FDA to withdraw the drug from the market. However, the FDA first decided to do a collaborative study designed to document whether there was truly an increase in the risk of hemorrhagic stroke in patients using PPA. This certainly took the immedieate pressure off the FDA to remove it. The investigation became known as the Yale Study.

Yale Study Results

In May of 2000, the Yale group reported these findings to the FDA:

> Women between the ages of 17 and 49 were 15 times more likely to suffer a hemorrhagic stroke if they were taking PPA (an estimated 200 to 500 hemorrhagic strokes occur each year in patients in this age group).
>
> Since consumers bought approximately six billion doses of PPA during the previous year, researchers anticipated published reports of the estimated number of patients suffering a stroke to be much higher than previously thought.

The FDA ordered that all over-the-counter manufacturers remove PPA from their products.[9]

Drug manufacturers were well prepared and positioned for the FDA's warning and withdrawal of PPA from the market. Within a matter of days after products containing PPA were recalled, the drug manufacturers substituted products containing the comparable, but much safer drug *pseudoephedrine*. These new products with similar labeling began appearing on the shelves within a few weeks of the FDA's advisory.

> How many more over-the-counter drugs possess potentially dangerous side effects? More than we would like to believe.

This story of an over-the-counter drug that had been on the market for more than six decades shows how difficult it really is to determine the safety of medications. If it were not for the fact that these strokes were occurring in very young women like Katie, we still would not realize that PPA could seriously injure people. Many severe adverse drug reactions occur in normal disease processes. Problems with PPA finally became apparent through specific case reports, journal articles, and the focus of the Yale Study. How many more over-the-counter drugs possess potentially dangerous side effects? More than we would like to believe.

Self-Medicated Society

Not only are we an overmedicated society, we are a self-medicated one. It's true, physicians are prescribing more drugs than ever before, but not only is the pharmaceutical industry effective in advertising prescription medications, it has overwhelmingly persuaded the American public to buy tons of over-the-counter medications.

Furthermore, the FDA continues to make more and more drugs available without prescription. Medications I once prescribed for my patients can now be purchased over the counter, such as ibuprofen, Naproxen, Tagamet, Pepcid, and Rogaine. We can be certain that in the years to come, this trend will continue.

We consumers usually consider a drug's change of status from prescription to over-the-counter as a positive move, because then we can buy our drug without seeing the doctor first, and it usually becomes available at a significantly lower cost. Still, keep in mind that if your insurance pays for medication, it typically doesn't cover over-the-counter drugs.

Here's another twist as to why some drugs end up becoming available over the counter: Presently lawsuits are pending between health insurance companies and manufacturers of some nonsedating antihistamine drugs, which have been notoriously expensive. This at first may seem odd. But the fact is, if these drugs become available over the counter, the insurance companies no longer have to pay for them. Now isn't that a switch in strategy? In fact, Claritin is now the first non-sedating antihistamine that is over the counter. I am sure others will follow.

Self-Care Guidelines/Drug-to-Drug Interactions

After reading Chapter 8 you are aware that drugs may interact with one another and cause dangerous side effects. Many people, however, still do not consider over-the-counter medication and herbal therapies "true" drugs. After reading this book you will become a wiser consumer with heightened awareness of the drugs you are combining.

Here are several guidelines for minimizing your risk of developing a serious adverse drug reaction to over-the-counter medications:

- Remember that over-the-counter medications are drugs and have inherent risks of adverse drug reactions like any prescription medication.
- Be aware of the "active ingredients" contained in each of the over-the-counter drugs you are taking. The box or container of your medication plainly notes these ingredients.
- Read the directions carefully for exactly how and how much you should take of your medication, especially if it is in liquid form.
- Read all the information that appears on the OTC label and package insert.
- Become familiar with medical conditions that are contraindicated (medical situations where this drug should not be taken) when taking each medication. For example, there are over-the-counter drugs that should not be taken if you suffer from illnesses such as hypertension, glaucoma, heart disease, or ulcer disease. You need to avoid these medications, and consult your physician.
- Inform your physician of any over-the-counter medications you may be taking on a routine basis.
- Know which drugs may interact with your particular over-the-counter medication.
- Consult your pharmacist anytime you have questions about what you might need to take.
- If your symptoms do not improve within a few days, make an appointment to see your personal physician. After all, you have been self-diagnosing and self-medicating; there is a possibility you made the wrong diagnosis and are taking the wrong kind of medication.

Hazel's Story

Hazel was thankful and never took for granted her excellent health. At age seventy-eight, she shared a busy life with her four children and nine beautiful grandchildren. She loved kids and except for the eight years she stayed home with her own children, she'd taught school. Even after retiring, she continued volunteering as a classroom aid at the elementary school in her neighborhood. She had taught hundreds of children to read!

Only once had Hazel been hospitalized other than when she was birthing children. At age forty-four she came down with a terrible bout of pneumonia, but since then she hadn't been ill. Her annual checkups were good, and she never took medication other than an occasional aspirin.

Just recently she'd begun developing a significant amount of stiffness in her hands and knees and occasionally in her left hip. In the mornings she was especially stiff, and her fingers even felt a little swollen. As the day progressed, she felt better and was able to do almost everything she wanted. As the months went along, however, and especially during the spring, she began having some very difficult days.

At first Hazel just attributed her stiffness to old age and didn't say anything. Stubborn and independent, she didn't want her kids fussing over her. Then one morning while her friend Patty was over for a cup of coffee, Patty told Hazel that she, too, was having similar problems and that she'd started taking naproxen. It did wonders for her, and she could get it over the counter without a prescription. She suggested that her friend try it.

Hazel went down to her local drugstore and found a long shelf full of arthritis medication, including aspirin, acetimenophen, ibuprofen, and naproxen. She decided to go with the generic naproxen, since it was less expensive and it seemed to be the same thing.

She looked at the directions for how to take the medication but admitted later she really didn't carefully look at the other information. After taking two 220 mg naproxen both morning and night for a couple of weeks, Hazel began feeling marked improvement in both her hands and knees. She was able to do chores and needlepoint projects that she'd had to put aside in the past year or two. When she forgot her medication, the pain would come back and remind her to take it.

Things were going well for Hazel except for the fact that she had developed some nausea and vague abdominal pain. She felt that she must have eaten something that didn't agree with her. The feeling would subside for a few days or so and then return with a vengeance. She'd never had stomach problems before, and it never even crossed her mind that the culprit could be the medication she was taking.

In early June Hazel started to feel weak and a little achy all over. She really thought she was coming down with the flu or something and was barely able to do her housecleaning. She hated having to call her daughter to cancel baby-sitting for the next few days, but her symptoms got worse. She began feeling light-headed and even thought she was going to pass out a time or two.

Finally, at the bidding of her daughter, she called her doctor and scheduled an appointment for later in the week. Hazel hoped she could make it that long. When she arrived at her physician's office, he noticed right away that his patient was pale and extremely weak. He asked if she had noted any changes in her stool color or evidence of bleeding anywhere.

Hazel did remember that her stools had become very dark but dismissed it, thinking she had probably eaten something different. Her doctor did a rectal exam and drew a blood count. He then left the exam room, telling Hazel he would be right back once he had the lab test results.

When the physician came back into the exam room, he was obviously disturbed. Hazel's hemoglobin was down to 5.7 (normal is greater than 13.5), and her stools tested positive for blood. He had been seeing Hazel for years, and her results came as a total surprise. He couldn't even remember ever writing her a prescription. He asked if she'd been taking any medication. At first Hazel said that she wasn't but then remembered her over-the-counter arthritis medication. When she told him that she had been taking naproxen off and on for the past few months, he began asking her more specific details about her stomach discomfort. After learning all the details about Hazel's complaints, he explained that she was most likely bleeding from her stomach as a result of the naproxen. "We need to get you to the hospital immediately," he said.

While Hazel was in the doctor's office, she collapsed to the floor.

The doctor called for an ambulance and then the emergency room, alerting them that Hazel was en route and that she would need a blood transfusion upon arrival.

By the time Hazel reached the hospital, her blood pressure had dropped to 60/40. She was cold and clammy in spite of the fact she was already receiving intravenous normal saline. The ER doctor drew blood so that he could type and cross-match her for blood, knowing that it would take at least forty-five minutes to an hour before the blood would be available. He added some plasma expander to her IV to improve her blood pressure and quickly called the GI specialist.

Hazel's condition steadily grew worse. When the GI specialist arrived in the ER, he decided to take her directly down to the endoscopy section of the hospital in order to perform an emergency scoping of her stomach. He hoped he could stop the bleeding. They would give her the blood as soon as it was available.

During the procedure, the GI specialist noted that her entire stomach was oozing blood, but there were one or two places where it seemed to be the heaviest. He cauterized these two areas and flushed Hazel's stomach with a solution he hoped would help stop the bleeding. The donated blood finally arrived, and they started pumping it into her as fast as they could.

Although many patients do not survive such an ordeal, Hazel was fortunate to recover nicely and was able to leave the hospital a week later. However, over 16,000 patients each year die from the use of prescription and over-the-counter nonsteroidal anti-inflammatories (NSAIDS).[10]

———

More than one hundred thousand hospital admissions last year were due to GI bleeding from nonsteroidal anti-inflammatory agents alone, and people purchased most of them over the counter. It is also estimated that nearly sixteen thousand patients died from complications of a GI bleed.[11]

The frightening story you have just read is occurring over and over again.

Two independent studies interviewed patients who were admitted to the hospital for this very problem. Researchers found that more than 35 percent of those interviewed did not realize their medications could cause stomach ulcers and GI bleeding. Most patients told the interviewers that neither their doctors nor pharmacists had warned them about this common complication.[12]

> Most patients told the interviewers that neither their doctors nor pharmacists had warned them about this common complication.

Researchers believe without a doubt that most victims could have avoided death if they simply had known to stop taking these medications at the very first sign of GI distress (stomach pain, nausea, bloating, black stools).[13]

———

Our growing culture of self-care carries with it freedom and much responsibility. Easy access does not ensure safety.

We must educate ourselves and our children about the inherent danger of all drugs. What example are you setting for your children? Become familiar with the drugs in your cabinets, and purge the ones you aren't sure of! Don't procrastinate in making decisions about over-the-counter medications until you are so ill you can hardly find the box. Do some research now. Some helpful guidelines and resources are provided at the end of this book.

Are you feeling ready to give up on drugs altogether and consider instead natural treatments? Wait. Before you visit your local health-food store, read the next chapter about the pharmaceutical properties in herbal therapies.

CHAPTER TWELVE

Herbal Therapies

HOME REMEDIES CREATED FROM HERBS ARE GREAT FUN TO read about and even more fun to hear described by a grandparent or great-aunt while you're perched next to a potbellied stove or sitting on a porch swing. Many old concoctions are truly effective, and those who tell about them often spin their stories with folklore and family history. You usually don't hear about a good old remedy without hearing also about a heroic deed and how folks pulled through a miserable crisis.

Have you ever wondered if we wouldn't all be better off going back to simpler times . . . all "natural"? My grandmother was a firm believer in natural home remedies and herbal therapies. In fact, when I announced that I had been accepted into medical school, she pulled out a large, hardbound book filled with natural cures and gave it to me. At the time, I was a bit offended. Though I graciously accepted it, I stashed it with my belongings to be packed away in storage. I didn't have time for what I considered outdated old-wives' stuff. I was off to study the latest breakthroughs in medicine!

I have since dusted off that big old book and been amazed by its many effective antidotes. I fondly remember the day I left for medical school. My grandma pulled me close to share her secret for excellent health—garlic. She ate raw garlic harvested from her lovely vegetable garden every day of her adult life. When I reflect back on her simple lifestyle as a farmer's wife who relied on many household cures, I can't help but wonder if this wasn't the reason she lived a robust life to age ninety-four—then died of old age. Need I say I now take my daily dose of garlic?

Home Remedies

For Itchy Skin: Oatmeal

Soaking in an oatmeal bath can be great for soothing skin irritations, including the itch of poison ivy and poison oak, dryness, bee stings, hives, insect bites, and sunburn.

Fill your tub with tepid water and add one to two cups of oatmeal. Oatmeal will stop the itching, and it's very soothing to the skin.

For Bladder Infections: Cranberry Juice

Doctors often recommend drinking lots of fluids to help prevent painful bladder infections, because fluid dilutes the urine and flushes out the bacteria. But there's something about cranberry juice that makes it even more effective.

Cranberry juice works because it prevents the bacteria that cause the infection from sticking to the lining of the urinary tract. If you're prone to these infections, drink eight ounces of cranberry juice every day to lower your risk.

For Nausea: Ginger

Ginger can do more than just add zip to cakes and cookies; the herb, in tablet form, can also help relieve nausea.

Ginger may also help prevent motion sickness. Try drinking a cup of ginger tea thirty minutes before your next trip. To make the tea: Take a piece of fresh ginger about the size of your knuckle. Skin and dice it, and put it in a mug with a little brown sugar. Pour boiling water over the mixture and steep for five minutes. If you don't have fresh ginger, use a half-teaspoon of the powdered variety.

Two Different Worlds—or Not

As a traditional physician, I hadn't spent much time at the health-food store. But my wife was terribly ill and nothing I had prescribed would make her better. On the other hand, she had made some amazing improvements by simply taking some nutritional supplements. I then decided to venture into a small health-food store to see if I could put together a similar mixture of supplements.

With more than a little hesitation, I pushed open the door, trying my best to look like I frequented places like these. A small woman nodded in my direction. She and several other shoppers looked especially hungry to me in their baggy clothes and Birkenstocks. They all browsed the aisles, seeming to know what they were looking for.

In a sweeping glance I discovered organic fruit and veggies, eggs, tofu, and soy milk on one side, big barrels of whey powder and soy products, carob balls, lentils in the raw, and whole-wheat pasta in the back, and packaged stuff down the middle. Trying to ignore the unfamiliar aromas, I then spotted several rows of shelves loaded with every different herb combination you might imagine.

Aha, just what I need. Now if I could just find a shopping cart. As if sensing my need, the cashier silently pointed to a pile of burlap shoulder bags over by the door. Two hours and $358 later, I left with a small bag (recycled, of course) of natural products—sure to make my wife feel better. Needless to say, I have returned to the nutritional supplements that initially helped her. They are not only better, but easier to take and less expensive at around $40.00 per month.

We tend to think of herbs and synthetic drugs as an either/or paradigm— traditional or alternative. We anticipate either walking into a brightly lit room smelling of antiseptic, bracing ourselves for a cotton swab, or the opposite extreme: entering a dim room filled with large plants, wind chimes, and a water fountain trickling in the corner. Realistically, however, herbs and synthetic drugs are not worlds apart. They actually originate on the same continuum.

For those who desire to be proactive in protecting their health by the most natural means, it is difficult to know where to start or what the end result should be. Have you ever wondered how or why remedies, herbs, and nutritional supplements line shelves separate from pharmaceutical drugs? After all, the majority of humanity—for the majority of human history—has relied on the medicinal qualities of plants and therapies passed down from one generation to the next. What changed?

I will help explain this by answering these questions:

1. What is a natural nutrient (nutritional supplement)?
2. What are herbs (natural drugs that come from nature but have pharmaceutical properties)?
3. What is a synthetic drug?

Nutritional Supplementation

Let me clarify an important distinction right away: nutritional supplements such as Vitamin A, C, and E are not drugs but natural nutrients we should be getting from our foods. But because of depleted soils, early harvesting, hybrids, added pesticides, and food-storage techniques, our foods no longer provide all the necessary vitamins and minerals. Oxidative stress is the root cause of more than seventy chronic degenerative diseases. Oxidative stress is the damage to our bodies caused by excessive free radicals, or what are otherwise known as charged oxygen molecules. The very same oxidation process that causes a cut apple to turn brown or iron to rust is literally the cause of most of our chronic degenerative diseases like heart disease, cancer, stroke, diabetes, arthritis, Alzheimer's dementia, etc.

The best defense against developing such diseases as heart disease, cancer, stroke, and Alzheimer's dementia is by enhancing our bodies' natural defenses by taking nutritional supplements. Through supplementation we are now able to obtain these nutrients at optimal levels. I have written extensively about this in my book *What Your Doctor Doesn't Know About Nutritional Medicine May Be Killing You* (Thomas Nelson Publishers, 2002).

Herbs/Herbal Therapy

We are seeing amazing growth in the use of *herbal therapies*—most of them combine ten to twenty different herbs. One in three people in the United States used at least one form of alternative medicine in 1990. By 1997, people in the U.S. spent $3.24 billion annually for herbal therapies. Many countries use herbs exclusively and prefer them to synthetic medications. In Germany, estimates show that its citizens spend more than $4 billion on herbs each year.[1]

There is a definite misconception among consumers when it comes to herbs. A national survey reported that the majority of herb users interviewed believed that herbs were as effective, safe, and cost-efficient as nonherbal remedies. Their false belief in the safety of these herbs is potentially dangerous. Nutritional supplements are used in normal enzymatic reactions throughout the body; herbs actually have a drug effect. They block certain natural enzymatic reactions to create a therapeutic effect. For example, St. John's wort is basically half-strength Prozac. Because herbs are not as potent as synthetic prescription medication, they have fewer side effects. But because they have a drug effect in the body, they do have side effects.

> Because herbs are not as potent as synthetic prescription medication, they have fewer side effects. But because they have a drug effect in the body, they do have side effects.

Synthetic Drugs

Manufacturers produce synthetic (pharmaceutical) drugs in a lab. These also block a natural enzymatic reaction in the body in order to create a therapeutic effect—however, they are much stronger than herbs. Until now, this entire book has focused on the development and potential complications of pharmaceutical drugs. Please know, however, the pharmaceutical industry has in no way ignored herbal or natural drugs. Pharmacognosy, the study of natural drugs and their constituents, plays a major role in the current development of new drugs. Many of our medications are the result of enhancing the pharmaceutical effect of herbal drugs as a means of developing more potent drug therapies. In fact, over the past twenty-five years, approximately 25 percent of all prescription drugs in the United States have contained active constituents obtained from plants.[2]

Over the past eight years, I have personally become more involved with what I call complementary medicine. After extensively researching the medical literature, I realize the health benefits my patients can receive by consuming high-quality, complete, and balanced nutritional supplements. Therefore I encourage my patients to adopt healthy lifestyles, which should include a healthy diet, a modest exercise program, and nutritional supplementation (see Chapter 14 for more details). I encourage my patients to make these healthy lifestyle changes to help improve their blood pressure, lower their cholesterol, and decrease their risk of diabetes and heart disease. The medical literature strongly supports this approach, and this allows me to use medication as a last resort rather than a first choice.

Years ago my wife, Liz, began to feel tired frequently. It was easy enough to chalk it up to the demands of being a wife and a mother of three children under the age of four. However, by the time we reached our fifteenth wedding anniversary, her total body pain and severe fatigue affected every decision in our life. In spite of the nine different medications she was taking for her pain, allergies, recurrent sinusitis, and bronchitis, she was doing poorly. When a friend introduced her to some potent nutritional supplements, I was able to see for myself her miraculous improvement.

Within months, the sparkle returned to my wife's eyes. She was able to again ride her horses and seemed to have completely renewed strength and joy. She was no longer taking any medications, because she did not have a need for them. I had always dismissed vitamin supplementation as simply the ingredients for "expensive urine." This experience with my wife proved to be the launching pad for an eight-year quest to learn more about nutritional medicine, which I have come to realize is really just "true" preventive medicine.

I fully realize the impact of the disappointment many patients have with traditional medicine. As a result, a shift to alternative healing methods and a renewed interest in herbal therapies has taken place. But the medicinal qualities of herbs are not something we can treat lightly. Most people consider all herbs to be "natural" and therefore, perfectly safe. The most important thing you need to remember here is that herbs, unlike vitamins, are natural drugs . . . but they are still drugs.

> The most important thing you need to remember here is that herbs, unlike vitamins, are natural drugs . . . but they are still drugs.

All About Herbs

The Synthetic/Herbal Split

The Kefauver-Harris legislation of 1962 required pharmaceutical companies to prove their products to be safe and effective before they could market them. When these laws were enacted, some pharmaceutical companies complied with the regulations and provided scientific evidence of the safety and efficacy of their products. Others, however, discontinued manufacturing some of their products because the cost of complying was too high.

Many of the herbal medications were the ones that fell by the wayside. Since they were natural medications, the manufacturers could not patent them, nor could the FDA regulate them. Therefore, some manufacturers began marketing herbal medicines as "nutritional supplements"—a legislative loophole that allowed products with no proven efficacy to be sold as long as the manufacturers made no claims on the product label.

The Dietary Supplement Health and Education Act of 1994 (DSHEA) also classified herbs as nutritional supplements. Again, the labeling of dietary supplements could carry no claims of therapeutic benefit. Therefore, manufacturers had to market herbs as benefiting a natural body function and not as a treatment for a disease process. Under this legislation, a manufacturer could claim that St. John's wort could improve one's mood but could not claim that it could help depression. Ginseng provides another example: its makers could promote it as helping give the body energy but not as a treatment for chronic fatigue.

If a manufacturer does make a claim on the product label, it must add, "This statement has not been evaluated by the FDA. This product is not intended to diagnose, treat, cure, or prevent any disease." DSHEA allows the FDA the power to remove a supplement from the market only when it is found to have dangerous side effects.

Herbs most definitely have a pharmaceutical effect in the body. Even though the government regards them as "nutritional supplements," you must scrutinize them as drugs. This major dilemma has resulted because we do not have good, well-controlled studies to elicit their safety and effectiveness. Herbal manufacturers simply do not have monetary incentives to finance such studies. Instead, they rely on selling their products by anecdotal evidence and word-of-mouth testimonies.

Most of the evidence of the effectiveness and safety of herbal medicines comes from Germany. In 1978, the German Federal Health Agency established German Commission E, a regulatory body that evaluates the safety and efficacy of herbs. This commission bases its decisions on clinical trials, cases, and all the other scientific information it can gather. Because the German Commission E has published more than 320 monographs (written details of the pharmaceutical effects of these herbs) based on these clinical trials since its inception, manufacturers can market herbs in Germany with drug claims. Many physicians in that country prescribe herbal remedies for their patients with the luxury of knowing their manufacturers must follow strict quality controls.

No Quality Control in America

We have no such standard of quality control with the production of herbal medicines in the United States. Without this control we have absolutely no assurance that the tablet contains what the bottle claims it does. No organization or government agency certifies the accuracy of herb labels. This lack of safeguarding results in two major flaws: First, independent studies show that many herb products don't contain any active ingredients, or they contain only trace amounts. Second, they may actually contain too much of the active ingredient and place the patient in harm's way. Chemical analysis of commercially available herbs has demonstrated both of these problems.[3]

> We must give herbal plants more respect, and realize that they are potentially dangerous in and of themselves and also have the potential to interact with prescription drugs we may already be taking.

The basic problem with herbs is the fact that no one has thoroughly studied them, and no one fully understands the extent of their potential risks. The reporting system for adverse herbal effects is essentially nonexistent. We all know that drugs have a dark side, but when it comes to herbs we feel they are basically safe. We must give herbal plants more respect, and realize that they are potentially dangerous in and of themselves and also have the potential to interact with prescription drugs we may already be taking.[4]

Let me assure you that herbs carry risk and, in some cases, a substantial risk. Don't let the concept of "natural medicines" blind you.

Juan's Story

Juan was a twenty-five-year-old manager of a busy retail business. He liked participating in community sport leagues and especially liked lifting weights. After being a member of a local gym for several years, he considered competing and began a serious workout program. A trainer at the exercise facility encouraged him to take a natural herbal product to help him have a better workout. Juan gladly tried the product and asked the trainer what was in it. He said it was basically caffeine and ephedra, a natural herb that would boost energy. For the next year, Juan continued to work out, using ephedra with no problems. His body looked amazing, and soon he had met the love of his life.

The next year Juan married Christina, and a year and a half later they were blessed with a beautiful baby girl. Being a husband, father, and the manager of a very successful business began to take a toll on Juan. He gained some weight and found that his stressful lifestyle, which included getting up at 5:00 A.M. after waking several times in the night to a crying baby, was causing him fatigue. Hoping to boost his energy, he decided to start taking the caffeine and ephedra product again, which he had quit taking about nine months earlier. The young father was working yet another long, arduous day and had gone through the evening without eating. He was tired and wanted to go home, but he needed to stay and close some accounts before the end of the fiscal period. He didn't dare nod off while doing the detailed financial work, so he decided to take his regular dose of the ephedra. This time, however, things turned out differently.

Christina recalls Juan calling her about 9:00 P.M. and telling her that he didn't feel good. He had a headache and was having trouble thinking. She encouraged him to just come home and rest; he could have his assistant finish the paperwork. Juan told her he'd just tough it out. He didn't want to risk any mistakes.

Less than thirty minutes later he collapsed and started to have a grand mal seizure. The assistant manager called 911, and an ambulance took Juan directly to the ER. Then the assistant called Christina. When she arrived at the hospital, her husband was still having seizures. The CAT scan of the brain was negative, but the brain wave study (called an EEG) produced unbelievable results. Juan was in a continuous state of seizures called "status epilepticus."

The prolonged seizure kept Juan from breathing, so it compromised the oxygen supply to his brain. The EMT had inserted an endotracheal tube and had been artificially ventilating Juan since he had arrived at

Juan's place of business. But it had taken the medics twelve to fifteen minutes to arrive and another five minutes to establish an airway. The neurologist explained to Christina that Juan could have suffered brain damage because of lack of oxygen. The only option now to stop these seizures was to administer a heavy sedating medication, which would essentially place him in a coma.

Day after day, Christina and her daughter went to visit Juan in the hospital. It was horrible seeing him on a respirator and comatose. Months passed, and the doctors began to have little hope of his survival. They explained to Christina that they believed the seizures were a result of the natural herb combination of caffeine and ephedra that Juan had been taking. The neurologist had seen this same reaction twice before in her career. She said that even if Juan did manage to survive, he would most likely sustain significant brain damage.

After three months the EEG had settled down enough that the neurologist felt she could take her patient off the sedation and try to wake him up. Juan came off the ventilator without any problems and remained seizure-free with the help of medication. Sadly, he had sustained major hypoxic (lack of oxygen) brain damage.

For weeks Christina prayed for the complete recovery of her husband. She watched for any sign of improvement, but she saw little. After the fourth month, the neurologist began to make arrangements for Juan to go home. She informed Christina that her husband had recovered as much as he would. She might notice some slight changes over the next several months, but she should not expect much.

Today Juan has the mental capacity of about a three- or-four-year-old child. He requires total care with no change in sight. This tragic outcome was the result of his taking a natural herb just to get a boost of energy.

Juan's is not an isolated case. The FDA has received reports of more than forty deaths and hundreds of serious injuries in patients using herbal products containing ephedra. It is a popular product found in many natural herbal weight-loss and energy-boosting products. Adding caffeine to the ephedra accentuates the adverse side effects of increased heart rate and blood pressure and has led to strokes, heart attacks, and seizures in numerous individuals.[5]

The FDA has issued warnings about the amount of ephedra that consumers should use. These state that you should take no more than 8 mg "per serving" and never exceed 25 mg for the entire day. (It warns that patients with heart disease, hypertension, kidney disease, or a previous stroke should avoid this nutrient altogether.)[6] This recommendation seems ridiculous, though, in an industry with no quality control. How would one actually know how much ephedra is in the herb he is taking?

Dangerous Herbs

Several herbs are known to have harmful side effects for the user. These risks often remain undisclosed to herb users even though they have been reported in the medical literature. Like the doctors who don't inform their patients of known side effects found in the medical literature, many herbalists and health food store workers are either not aware of the literature and the reports, or simply fail to inform the buyer. Though we've yet to discover many health risks related to herbs, we need to look carefully at some of the documented problems in order to keep a realistic perspective on herbal therapies.

Some herbs contain dangerous products called pyrrolizidine alkaloids, which are known to cause liver damage while leading to cancer in animals; for example: borage (*Borago officinalis*), coltsfoot (*Tussilago farfar*), comfrey (*Symphytum* species), and life root (*Senecio aureus*).[7]

The German Federal Health Agency has established regulations on the amount of pyrrolizidine alkaloids that their manufacturers may place in these herbs. Germany, however, does require quality control and so actually regulates these amounts. In the United States, we really do not have a clue how many pyrrolizidine alkaloids are in our products.

Other products are also of concern. Researchers have found that the safrole in sassafras (*Sassafras albidum*) and cis–isoasarone in calamus (*Acorus calamus*) have carcinogenic potential in animals in U.S. studies.[8] Since we don't have human studies using herbs in the U.S., we should at least be concerned about the results of animal studies.

There are human case reports of jaundice, fatigue, severe itching, elevated liver enzymes, and even liver failure in patients taking chaparral (*Larrea tridentata*), germander (*Teucrium chamaidrys*), and life root (*Senecio aureus*).[9] These reactions have been reported within three weeks of patients' taking these herbs, but they also may not manifest themselves for months.[10]

Did you know licorice root (*Glycyrrhiza glabra*) has the potential to cause serious complications? When a person uses licorice root at high doses over a long period of time, he may experience headache, fatigue, water retention, low potassium, hypertension, and cardiac arrest. Glycyrrhizin, the active ingredient in licorice root, can stimulate the release of an adrenal hormone called aldosterone. This may lead to the retention of sodium, loss of potassium, and fluid retention; and over time this can cause high blood pressure, increasing heart failure, and other cardiac problems.[11] The German Commission E recommends that people use licorice no longer than four to six weeks.[12]

Because of these potential problems, patients who have kidney disease, liver disease, heart disease, or who are pregnant should not use licorice.[13]

Herbal Interactions with Drugs

Patients must realize that because herbs are drugs, they can accentuate the pharmaceutical drugs a physician prescribes. As a physician, this is my greatest concern. Studies reveal that three out of four patients will not communicate to their doctors that they are taking an herb or group of herbs.[14]

The best illustration of this point is St. John's wort. Many people take St. John's wort to treat their depression, because it works similarly to the antidepressants physicians prescribe, such as Paxil, Prozac, Zoloft, and Effexor. As I've said before, patients are self-medicating and self-treating more now than ever before. Only when their symptoms do not improve do they typically consult their physician. Often patients are too embarrassed to tell their physician that they've been trying to treat their depression on their own. Unknowing, the physician will go ahead and prescribe an antidepressant, and send the patient on his or her way.

The problem? Most patients do not know they should not take both St. John's wort and an antidepressant together. After all, they reason, St. John's wort is "natural," right? The thought of harm never crosses their minds. By itself, St. John's wort is relatively safe if the manufacturer has produced a quality product. But when a person combines herbal therapy with a pharmaceutical antidepressant, he or she may experience a serious adverse drug reaction. This occurs because two drugs are being combined—just like any other drug interaction. The combined pharmaceutical effect may create difficulties that neither one would cause when used alone.

As when a physician uses Prozac and Zoloft together, the drugs will actually enhance each other's effect in the body, possibly leading to serotonin syndrome (serotonin excess), especially if the person combines the St. John's wort with an MAO inhibitor (Nardil or Parnate). Both St. John's wort and the antidepressants increase the levels of serotonin, which improves the patient's depression. Yet too much serotonin can create a syndrome of agitation, irritability, headache, and even confusion.[15]

As well, St. John's wort in combination with black cohosh may be contraindicated, which means it should not be used during pregnancy and lactation due to potential uterine stimulation, which could lead to a miscarriage.[16]

Ginkgo biloba has become a popular herb for a wide variety of medical problems, the most common being hardening of the arteries. Several studies have shown that *Ginkgo biloba* helps increase the circulation of blood in the brain and extremities. Many herbalists and researchers believe it improves one's ability to think and boosts stamina as a result of this increased blood flow. But *Ginkgo biloba* has an additional effect of thinning the blood, which can lead to serious complications if a person is also taking aspirin or Coumadin.[17]

Many herbs that patients use work very similarly to prescription sedatives such as Ativan, Xanax, and Librium. The two most common herbs are valerian root and Kava Kava. Who is making you aware that when you combine either of these herbs with a prescription sedative, the combination may cause increased sedation and can lead to more serious problems than when you use the drugs separately?[18]

The use of hawthorn and the drug digoxin (digitalis) has also brought about concern. They have similar pharmaceutical effects on the heart and can potentially lead to complications when used together.[19] Licorice can also accentuate the loss of potassium when combined with common prescription diuretics like hydrochlorothiazide, Lasix, and Bumex. People generally use horsetail (*Equisetum arvense*), celery seed (*Apium graveolens*), dandelion leaf (*Taraxacum officinale*), and elder flower (*Sambucus nigra*) as natural diuretics, which rid the body of excess fluids.[20] But when a person combines these with prescription diuretics, he faces a significant potential for electrolyte abnormalities (sodium, potassium, and chloride).[21]

As you can see, herb and drug interactions pose a very real threat of producing serious adverse drug reactions. Table 1, on the following page, summarizes some of the most common interactions of herb and drug interactions. This is by no means an exhaustive list.

I personally feel that some natural therapies are safer and in some ways more effective than traditional medication. For example, I recommend that my patients try glucosamine sulfate for their arthritis while restricting their use of nonsteroidal anti-inflammatories (NSAIDS). Because of my new attitude toward supplements and herbal therapies, many people now consult me for advice on alternative therapies. I am still a physician, and I prescribe my share of medication; however, I hold firm to the belief that we should always use medication as a last resort and not as a first choice.

Many people take a hunt-and-peck approach to herbal treatments. If you are taking herbs or are seriously considering them, make your decision carefully and seriously. Know what you are dealing with. Please refer to the resource section at the end of the book, where I list several books on herbs that may prove to be helpful. Above all, know that when you choose to start taking an herb or group of herbs, you are actually using drugs. Respect this truth and have the courage to inform your doctor of *everything* you are taking.

Table 1

Common Herb/Drug Interactions	
Herb/Drug	**Interaction**
Licorice root/diuretics	Increases the loss of potassium
Ephedra/antihypertension medication	Increases blood pressure—may require increasing medication
Ginkgo biloba, ginseng, chamomile, red clover, garlic/Coumadin	Increases the blood-thinning effect of Coumadin
Valerian root, Kava Kava/ tranquilizers (Ativan, Xanax, Librium, Valium)	Accentuates the sedative effect of these tranquilizers and may lead to increased dependence
Horsetail, celery seed, dandelion leaf, elder flower/diuretics (Lasix, hydrochlorathiazide, Bumex)	Increases the risk of fluid and electrolyte abnormalities (potassium, sodium, and chloride)
St. John's wort/antidepressant medication (Prozac, Paxil, Zoloft)	Increases the effect of these drugs and can accentuate the adverse side effects
Hawthorn/digitalis (digoxin)	Accentuates the pharmacological action on the heart

CHAPTER THIRTEEN

Protecting Yourself

As I mentioned in the introduction, if I had written a book called *Death by Cancer* or *Death by Heart Attack,* people would nod knowingly with appreciation and hope for a broader understanding of these threatening diseases. But the title of this book, *Death by Prescription,* has caught some people off guard and has infuriated others. Why the display of emotion? Medications have become all but sacred. To discuss negative aspects of prescription meds seems taboo or at least inappropriate.

I don't agree. I believe you have the right to be informed. Only then will you be emboldened and empowered to step in and team with your medical community to prevent a possible adverse-reaction tragedy.

Ordinary stories often speak profound truths. Looking back over my day, I can now chuckle, but the enfolding events were sobering at the time and illustrate well the message of this chapter.

I looked out my window this morning to see a crew of workers trimming hedges and trees and cutting the grass. *Looks real nice,* I thought to myself as I turned back to my desk. In a quick, unassuming glance, I had viewed inviting shades of green that professionals were neatly manicuring as they tended my medical office grounds. I felt relaxed knowing I didn't have to concern myself with the worries of their equipment, watering, planting, or pruning techniques. They were responsible for their area of expertise.

What I failed to notice was one employee digging a hole with the intent of planting a new tree. If I had looked a little more carefully, I might have seen this crew member aggressively digging right next to a power box. As you might anticipate, the diligent young fellow dug an impressive hole, but he also cut a line, which then shut down the power to the medical building, which then sent my day skidding on its head! A series of difficulties arose that will take weeks to straighten out.

It would have taken no more than five minutes to question the groundskeeper, but my subconscious led me to believe that he was doing his job; I had other concerns to tend to so I didn't really pay attention. As a result, the man cut a line, and I had to scramble in the dark to help my assistants reset appointments, make phone calls, care for patients who had already arrived, and yes, have a "chat" with the grounds crew. The hours ticked past and in the midst of the flurry, my secretary calmly reminded me of an important meeting scheduled to start any minute at an office twenty minutes across town. Yikes! If I hurried I could make it, even though I'd be late.

Making a mad dash to the parking lot, I slowed to a trot as I approached my parking space. *Where was my car?* Of course! Behind the utility truck, whose crew had come to repair the electrical line the grounds crew had downed. Where was the utility crew? All gone to lunch! Steaming, I walked back to my office to make yet another phone call. I began to feel like the brunt of a bad joke.

If you're smiling and shaking your head, you've experienced a day or two like mine. Someone or something beyond your control dropped the ball, and it started rolling in the wrong direction, gathering speed as it went. These scenarios are bound to happen, but when they happen in medicine, the damage can be irreparable.

Physicians and health-care providers spend countless hours and dollars teaching you how to avoid cancer, heart disease, strokes, and diabetes. But why don't they instruct you on how you can avoid suffering from a serious adverse drug reaction? We are, after all, health-care professionals and should be concerned about protecting our patients from *all* causes of death. I figure if adverse drug reactions to properly prescribed medications are the fourth leading cause of death in the United States (and when combined with medical errors, the third leading cause of death), physicians should be just as avid about trying to protect patients from death or injury from a drug as from cancer or heart disease. Especially when you realize that over half of these serious adverse drug reactions and subsequent deaths can and should be avoided.

The fact remains: the medical community isn't passionate about your protection against adverse drug reactions. Hundreds of studies and articles abound in our medical literature regarding the seriousness of this problem (I've listed many in the references section of this book). Physicians study the major side effects of medications in medical school, but rarely do they address the serious and far-reaching implications of the problem. Furthermore, physicians and hospitals aren't inclined to report adverse reactions, due to the overriding concern of medical/legal action and bad publicity for their institutions.

This means that you must become familiar with the potential problems of each and every drug you are taking. Even when your doctor or pharmacist informs you about *some* of the potential risks of the drugs you are about to take, you need to be proactive yourself to find out as much as you can about *all* the potential dangers of your medication.

Ultimately, you are the one who must take steps to protect yourself and your loved ones. Parents, learn this information to protect your children. Children, protect your aging parents. Grown children come into my office almost daily accompanying their aging parents in order to help their moms and dads better understand what medications they are taking and how they should be taking them.

I've designed this chapter to focus specifically on practical suggestions and ideas to help protect you and your family, starting today. Most of these suggestions come from my personal experience while practicing medicine; some also come from current research and medical journals.

Primary-Care Physician

I personally believe that each and every person should have a primary-care physician. If you do not presently have one, this is the first step to take in protecting yourself. Being in primary care may make me a little biased; still, I believe that finding a primary-care physician whom you can trust and openly communicate with is essential.

This physician could be a pediatrician, an internist, or a family physician. Do not, however, consider your local urgent-care center or emergency-care physician a primary-care physician. Most gynecologists are willing to fill the role of a primary-care physician, and some are very good. Others feel the need to use specialists when a problem arises that does not involve the reproductive organs. Spend time talking to different physicians in your community and find a good fit.

A primary-care physician is one whose main focus is to keep you healthy while trying to protect you from developing a serious illness. This health-care professional needs to be totally familiar with you and your health history. He or she should be the one performing your routine physicals and lab work and calling in a specialist when you need a diagnosis or treatment of a specific problem. Even if you require specialty care, the primary physician should be orchestrating your care by keeping records from all the specialists you may be seeing, so that at least one doctor is totally aware of the evaluations, problems, and drugs you are taking.

In case you have an acute or potential problem with any medication, the primary-care physician must be readily available to see you. He or she should review your drugs each time you make a visit in order to prevent a serious drug interaction. This may require contacting a specialist to discuss a problem with a prescription drug or treatment. In short, this physician is in charge of your or your family's health; choose him or her wisely.

Your Medication List

I am always amazed at how little patients know about the medications they are taking. Some patients can discuss a few of the names and the conditions for which their doctors prescribed the drugs; but many do not know any of the names or doses of the medications they are taking. Granted, one's primary-care physician should have a current list of all the patient's medications, but this does not always happen. The second most important step to protect yourself from an adverse drug reaction is to keep a running record of your medications.

I recommend that you type up an index card that fits in your purse or wallet with a complete, up-to-date list of all medications you are taking. This list should have the names and dosages of each drug, along with the name of the doctor who prescribed the medication. It is also helpful to have the actual date listed when you started taking the medication. See Figure 1 for an example of a medication card.

Sample medication card
Figure 1

Patient: Evans, Jane
Allergic to: Penicillin, Codeine

Drug	Dose	Frequency	Started	Physician
Cozaar	50 mg	Once Daily	9/1/00	Jones
Avandia	4 mg	Once Daily	2/1/01	Smith
Celebrex	200mg	Once Daily	6/1/01	Jones
Glucotrol	5 mg	Twice Daily	4/1/02	Smith
Antioxidant Tablet		Three times daily		
Mineral Tablet		Three times daily		
Phytoestrogen		Two times daily		

On this card or printout, you need to list all the drugs to which you have reacted. This does not necessarily mean an allergic reaction but should include medicines that you were not able to tolerate for *any* reason. If you had a bad side effect from a particular medicine, it should be on your list. For example, if you took Erythromycin at one time for a pharyngitis and developed severe abdominal pain, you need to record this on your card, even though this is more of a side effect of Erythromycin than a true allergic reaction. There will be times and situations that you want all this information readily available.

Your list should include any over-the-counter medications you are taking, even if only occasionally. Also include any nutritional supplements, vitamins, or herbs that you use. These may interact with your prescription medications, and it is important that your physician know exactly what you consume.

Protect your card (I suggest laminating it), and keep it current. This is perhaps the most important card you will carry and you should present it to every physician you see: urgent-care, emergency-room, and especially your primary-care physician. I can't tell you how helpful it is when patients come in with their lists of medications. When changing meds, I find it extremely helpful to see what drugs the patient has had problems with in the past.

Medical allergies, too, are essential for the doctor to know, but the availability of a list of drugs a patient has had difficulty taking in the past is even better. An awareness of the drugs you are taking gives the physician a chance to consider the possibility that your current complaints could indeed be coming from a reaction to one of your medications.

I have learned this is the first thing that health-care professionals should consider in a patient who has a new symptom or complaint. Frequently I am able to correlate the onset of symptoms to the time a patient started a particular medication. This is why it is important to document the date you actually begin taking a medication. If the medicine is not essential, it is easy to discontinue it for a while to see if the symptoms improve.

A good example of this happened to me last month. I had strained my elbow helping to lay stall mats in our horse barn. I couldn't play golf because of the pain, so I started taking a nonsteroidal anti-inflammatory. This helped my elbow, but a few days later I developed vertigo at night when I was lying down. I could not roll onto my left side without the room seeming to spin violently.

This went on for several days and then slowly went away. I didn't think much about it until one day my elbow began to give me more problems and I took more of the medication. That night I developed severe vertigo again. It then occurred to me that the spinning sensation was possibly a side effect of the medication I was taking. After all, I was writing a book on adverse drug reactions! Sure enough, a day or so after I quit taking the pain medication, the vertigo went away.

The important point to remember is that drugs can mimic disease and essentially cause any symptom you can name. A list of your current medications will help alert you and your physician to this possibility. Remember, reactions to medications are often delayed. They may not always occur right after you start a medication. For instance, if a drug is causing liver damage, it may take months before any symptoms develop. This leads to another very important point in helping protect yourself from a serious drug reaction: getting recommended blood work.

Recommended Blood Work

Many medications are known to cause potential harm to various organs of the body. These problems have become apparent during the preclinical trials or through postmarketing surveillance. Many of the warnings the FDA sends to physicians in "Dear Doctor" letters recommend that physicians do certain blood work to be sure a particular medication is not damaging the liver, thyroid, bone marrow, kidneys, and so forth. If your doctor recommends, for instance, that you have your liver function checked every two months for the first year you take a new med, there is a good reason for it. It is critical that you follow through with his recommendations. Your health and life may depend on it.

If you read information from the pharmacist, *Physicians' Desk Reference,* Internet, or a book about the particular medication you are taking, and it recommends certain blood work, it is imperative that you discuss this with your doctor—even if he has not recommended that these particular tests be done. One of the biggest problems patients face is a physician who is busy and difficult to pin down. Be assertive. Most doctors will agree to additional tests and proceed to schedule them.

If, on the other hand, your physician argues that these tests are not a necessity, never having seen any problems with the drug, his response is not adequate. Proper use of medications frequently involves evaluation of periodic blood work. This blood work is *your* protection. Find a doctor who will schedule the blood work the FDA and pharmaceutical companies recommend so that if you do have a reaction to the medication, you can discontinue it, hopefully before any permanent damage occurs.

Remember the Rezulin story (Chapter 5), when doctors were advised to get monthly liver tests during the first year a patient was taking the drug for diabetes? When the FDA researched how frequently physicians were administering these tests, less than 1 percent of patients were having their doctors check their liver function, even after the agency had sent out four separate warnings over a two-year period about potential liver damage the new drug could cause. Physicians must be made accountable in these situations, and there is no better person to do this than you, the patient.

Another good illustration of this problem is with the use of Mevacor, Zocor, Lipitor, or any other HMG-CoA reductase inhibitor ("statin" drug). All of these drugs can cause liver damage. Studies have shown damage occurring approximately 2 percent of the time. Because of this tendency, drug companies have encouraged physicians to get baseline liver functions with follow-up tests six and twelve weeks after starting the medication, and periodically thereafter. If tests detect no problems with elevated liver enzymes, the patient can continue taking the medication with liver functions checked periodically—for example, every three to six months—for as long as he uses the drug. Patients on these medications should also be aware of potential muscle damage.

Patient awareness of potential problems with any medication is critical. Reactions can be serious and life-threatening, as we saw with the drug Baycol. How do you learn about these potential problems? Patients and physicians must keep an open line of communication.

Patient/Physician Communication

Another important step in protecting yourself against a serious adverse drug reaction is learning to communicate effectively with your physician about the drugs he is prescribing. When your doctor has made a diagnosis of a particular disease or problem, he will usually want to start you on a medication right away. For example, if your doctor has determined that you have developed high blood pressure, he will prescribe you one of the hundred or so high blood pressure medications on the market today.

The doctor will usually tell you what category of medication this particular drug falls into, such as a diuretic, beta-blocker, ACE inhibitor, or calcium channel blocker. He will usually then explain how to take the medication: how many times a day and whether you should take it with or without food. He will also discuss the main side effects of the medication as well as the periodic blood work he recommends. In the case of a prescribed diuretic, the doctor may recommend periodic blood tests to be sure your potassium doesn't get too low.

I encourage patients to ask a few specific questions at this point. The first question should be whether there is any way you could avoid taking the medication in the first place. Are there any lifestyle changes that could improve your condition? Could you delay starting the medication and aggressively change some eating habits or maybe start an exercise program? If your physician tells you that you need to start the medication immediately, at least ask if lifestyle changes could help you improve enough that you could ease off the drug in the future.

If your physician determines that you definitely need to start taking the medication, ask whether this particular one could potentially cause a drug interaction with your other medications. He should know exactly what other medications you are taking. If not, pull out your medication card. This allows the physician the opportunity to address any potentially serious problem.

A confident physician will not find this question intimidating. He will simply review all the medications you are taking and respond. If he tells you to take the medication trusting that he knows what he is doing, red flags should pop up. Wrong answer! Having blind faith in your doctor and the medical system puts you in a precarious situation. Trust must be earned, not expected.

> Having blind faith in your doctor and the medical system puts you in a precarious situation. Trust must be earned, not expected.

The next question you need to ask your physician is, "What is the expected outcome from taking this particular medication?" The results may be assumed, but this is a very important question, because it forces the doctor to discuss with you his or her strategy for treating your health problem.

I can't tell you the number of times I've seen a physician start a blood pressure medication, then have the patient come back in a month or six weeks to see how he is doing. The blood pressure may not have responded to the initial medication, so he adds another medication to the first one. This is called *step therapy*. The doctor continues to add medication until the blood pressure comes under control.

This may be appropriate, but I've found over the years that patients will respond uniquely to different categories of high blood pressure medication. Studies serve as a guide as to which drug may work best for individuals. Your doctor needs to have an expected outcome or result from any medication before he writes a prescription. If you do not get that result, the physician should discontinue the present medication and try something different. It is important to remember that drugs are a lot like taxes—they are easy to add, but it takes an "act of Congress" to reduce or eliminate them.

There is a misconception among many physicians that if they warn their patients about possible side effects of any medication, the patients will surely develop them. In other words, the power of suggestion is at work, and the mind falsely perceives symptoms that the doctor warned about. This then becomes the basic excuse physicians use for not discussing side effects in detail.

Another misconception abounds. Physicians often anticipate (whether rightly or wrongly) that if patients read about all the potential problems with a particular drug, they will never take the medication. This may be true in some cases, but don't you as a consumer deserve complete and comprehensive information about the potential hazards of any medication you are considering? Now that you realize the entire process involved in the developing of the drug before it reaches the pharmacy shelf, I am sure you agree that the more you know about any drug, the better. This leads to the next step in protecting yourself from a serious adverse drug reaction.

Gathering More Detailed Information

Physicians simply do not have the time needed to go over medications in full detail. Most will kindly answer specific questions if you ask directly. But this is only the start of the information-gathering process. The next step involves having your prescription filled.

One of the most important changes you may need to make is to get *all* of your prescriptions filled at the same pharmacy. You may choose a local pharmacist or send your prescription into one of the many mail-order services available today. Either way, it is critical that you only use one source for all your

> It is important to remember that drugs are a lot like taxes—they are easy to add, but it takes an "act of Congress" to reduce or eliminate them.

medications. If this is not possible—for example, if you use a mail-in pharmacy for your chronic medications but a local pharmacy for your acute medications such as antibiotics—you need to be sure that both your local pharmacist and your mail-in pharmacist have records of all of the medications you are presently taking in their computer systems.

Many serious drug interactions involve the combination of an acute-care medication (medication used for acute treatment, like antibiotics, pain medication for an injury, etc.) with a long-term medication the patient has been taking for years. When patients took Erythromycin after having been on Seldane or Hismanal, the potential risk was sudden death.[1] This is why these drugs are now off the market. Be assured other drug interactions can potentially bring the same results.

You must also hold the pharmacist accountable. Choose a pharmacy where the pharmacist will actually talk to you. He or she, too, should go over any potential side effects and adverse reactions after checking the computer to be sure no drug interaction warnings came up as he recorded this new medication. Your pharmacist should then inform you of the best time(s) of the day to take the medication and confirm whether you should take it with or without food.

He or she should also include a drug information sheet with each new drug you purchase. Make a habit of reading this and understanding it thoroughly before ever starting a medication. Other great resources are also available to you as more complete references. *The Physicians' Desk Reference* (PDR), *The Pill Book, The Essential Guide to Prescription Drugs, The Complete Guide to Pills,* and *Worst Pills/Best Pills* (please refer to my resource section in the addendum of this book) provide warnings and recommended protocols such as routine blood work you may need.

———

I have always told my patients that if they feel any bad effects of the medication I prescribe, they should contact me or my staff immediately. You should not stop some drugs abruptly, however. In these situations, waiting to stop a medication until you can talk to your physician is not only wise but critical. Again, accessibility to your primary-care physician is a must. The physician or his or her partner should be available to you twenty-four hours a day, seven days a week. When you feel you may be reacting to a medication, you want to either call your doctor or see him or her that day.

Types of Drug Reactions

Allergic Reactions

The most common and recognizable drug reaction is a *pure* allergic reaction to medication. As you have learned throughout this book, drugs are synthetic (not natural), and the body considers them foreign invaders. Over time, a body's natural immune system may actually develop an immune response to a particular drug and create an allergic reaction. This usually does not happen the very first time you take a drug—for example, the first time you take penicillin. Rather, the body most often *develops* an allergy after repeated exposure to a particular drug, like penicillin.

A typical allergic reaction to a drug is welts that develop all over the body, commonly called *hives*, or in medical terms, *erythema multiforme*. Accompanying hives may be swelling of the tongue, lips, eyelids, or even the throat—which may be life-threatening because it potentially could close off your airway. Other more severe forms of allergic reactions involve swelling throughout the body, blister formation in the mouth and skin (Steven Johnson syndrome), shock, and even death.

At the first sign of a possible allergic reaction, you should stop the medication immediately (even if you aren't certain whether it is an allergic reaction or not). Although I have previously advised you to contact your physician first if you feel you may be reacting to a medication he or she has prescribed, in this particular situation (suspicious allergic reaction) it would not be wise to take another dose of your medication. However, you need to contact your physician as soon as possible or even go to an urgent-care center or emergency room. Again, allergic reactions can be serious and you may be placing yourself in harm's way to continue with the medication.

In the case of a severe allergic reaction—sometimes referred to as an *anaphylactic reaction*—you should go directly to your local emergency room. Time is of the essence. Physicians have the ability to stop allergic reactions and reverse their effects. If the reaction is happening very quickly, call 911 and have the emergency personnel sent to your home immediately.

Once you have developed an allergy to a medication, your body will react to this particular medication every time you take it. This is why it is critical for you to remember exactly which drugs you have reacted to previously. Another important fact is that many drugs are similar in composition or are members of a family of drugs, and you may potentially be allergic to every drug in that same category. For example, when you are allergic to penicillin, you need to avoid any drug that is similar, such as amoxicillin, ampicillin, methicillin, nafcillin, and piperacillin, to name just a few. If you are allergic to one of the nonsteroidal anti-inflammatory drugs such as ibuprofen (Motrin), you may also be allergic to Naproxen (Naprosen), Relafen, Clinoril, Daypro, or Voltaren.

> Once you have developed an allergy to a medication, your body will react to this particular medication every time you take it.

Expected Potential Reactions to Medications

Physicians are readily aware of and expect *potential* adverse drug reactions to every medication. This is because of the known pharmaceutical effects a particular drug may have in a patient. For example, if I prescribe a high blood pressure medication, I anticipate that the drug is going to lower the patient's blood pressure. But what happens if this particular medication actually lowers the blood pressure too much? The patient will develop hypotension (low blood pressure), dizziness, and may actually pass out. Often patients don't realize these are adverse drug reactions that their physicians can correct by adjusting or discontinuing the medication.

"Expected potential" adverse drug reactions occur when a patient is either especially sensitive to the pharmaceutical action of a particular drug or reacts during the period of time a physician is gradually increasing the dose of medication. It is common practice in medicine to increase the amount of medication a patient is taking (called *titrating* medication) until he or she reaches an expected or desired therapeutic response or the patient begins to develop an adverse drug reaction. If the latter occurs, the physician will then generally back off the dose, hoping the patient will tolerate it better. This is very common practice when treating high blood pressure, chronic pain, depression, and several other medical situations.

Complications may also arise in this category of drug reactions when a patient uses (or a doctor prescribes) two or more drugs that cause similar pharmaceutical effects in the body. For example, a physician may use a combination of medications that all lower the patient's blood pressure, such as a beta-blocker, a calcium channel blocker, and an ACE inhibitor along with a diuretic. All of these drugs may lower blood pressure, and the risk of developing hypotension or low blood pressure significantly increases. A physician may also add several drugs together that have a pharmaceutical effect of lowering the heart rate. Doctors sometimes use drugs such as digoxin, Verapamil (calcium channel blocker), and atenolol (a beta-blocker) in combination for various reasons. Every one of these drugs can slow down the patient's heart rate (in fact, it's not unusual to slow down the heart rate so much that the patient actually passes out).

Most precaution lists or discussions about a particular medication will detail all of these potential "expected reactions." This is why it is so important for patients to become familiar with the potential adverse side effects associated with the medications they are taking. Information, communication, and awareness are the keys of avoiding a serious adverse drug reaction.

Unexpected or Idiosyncratic Adverse Drug Reactions

Idiosyncratic drug reactions are rightly named because they make us feel like idiots—we don't expect them and they are impossible to explain. These are the most difficult and usually the most severe adverse drug reactions. Remember my patient in Chapter 1 who developed a severe and persistent cough from taking an ACE inhibitor for blood pressure? Another example of a bizarre idiosyncratic reaction is when a patient ruptured an Achilles tendon while taking a fluoroquinolone antibiotic for bronchitis. These reactions and several others are ones we physicians cannot anticipate. While most physicians are aware of the first two types of drug reactions, knowing all the unusual reactions a particular drug may cause is difficult at best.

You Need to Be the Authority When it Comes to *Your* Medication

The FDA intends that all preclinical trials and the postmarketing experience will discover these unusual and sometimes severe adverse drug reactions. The biggest challenge physicians face now is how to manage efficiently the voluminous amount of risk information that accumulates regarding a new drug as its manufacturer aggressively markets it to the public.

This is where you need to play a vital role in protecting your health and the health of your loved ones. The number of drugs you are presently taking or will take in the future is limited and hopefully quite manageable. If you make a concerted effort to learn everything you can about *your* particular drugs, you may avoid suffering or dying from an adverse drug reaction. Research thoroughly, and make the best clinical decisions for yourself. Even if your doctor is not fully informed of all the potential serious adverse drug reactions possible for the drug he prescribed for you—*you* need to know them. After all, it is your health and well-being you are trying to protect. Review the resource page in the back of the book, and find a couple of resources that work best for you. I personally feel that the Internet will give you the most complete and up-to-date information. However, some of the books can be great resources, especially if they are easy to use and understand.

My colleague and close personal friend, Dr. David Sabow, a retired local neurologist, used to tell his patients, "If you want to maintain your health, listen to your body and not your doctor." When it comes to adverse drug reactions, this could not be more appropriate. Never forget, we know only half of the adverse drug reactions at the time the

FDA first releases a drug. If a negative change is taking place in your body, and you are experiencing new symptoms, always think of a potential adverse drug reaction first—not last.

Adverse drug reactions can be very difficult to discern. But I have always trusted my patient's sensitivity to the fact that something just isn't right. This is when having specific information available about the drugs you are taking is very important. And if you've not read all the detailed information about your drug before, this would be a good time to start.

Wisdom in Choosing your Medications

I remember my professors in medical school advising me not to get my new medical information from a pharmaceutical representative. It is the farthest thing from unbiased information one can receive. Even though reps eagerly display recent clinical trials that have been reported in a peer-reviewed medical journal, and doctors often eagerly respond, you as the patient should still seek independent, unbiased information. The pharmaceutical company conducts or sponsors most of these trials.

> If a negative change is taking place in your body and you are experiencing new symptoms, always think of a potential adverse drug reaction first—not last.

In fact, the editors of the *New England Journal of Medicine*, the *Journal of the American Medical Association,* and the *British Lancet* have publicly announced their concern about the overall validity of many of such studies. These medical journals are now making a concerted effort to screen studies much more vigorously before printing them.[2]

If you consider the drugs we have reviewed in this book, the majority were recently released medications that arrived with great fanfare, hype, and marketing. But once these drugs were exposed to a large number of patients, adverse drug reports started rolling in. Because of the voluntary reporting system and biased analysis of these reports, most of these drugs were on the market for a significant length of time before the FDA forced their withdrawal.

I recommend that patients not take *any* drug that has not been out on the market for a minimum of five years. The voluntary reporting system will eventually work, and we will know the major side effects and problems with each and every drug. At least by using an older drug you can learn about all of the potential side effects and problems using that particular drug. Many of the Me-Too drugs that are being developed really offer only minor advantages, if any, over the older medications with which they are trying to compete. When your doctor reaches into his sample closet, you need to ask, "How long has this drug been on the market?" If he or she confidently states, "Oh, this is a new drug we're trying," politely ask if an older drug is available that would be just as effective.

> I recommend that patients not take *any* drug that has not been out on the market for a minimum of five years.

Free samples may seem economical, but you may find out later that you or your insurance company will end up paying the high price of the new drug as long as you are taking it. Older drugs are typically much less expensive and many are even generic. You can save as much as 20 to 80 percent each time you fill your prescription with an older drug.

(Table 1) Summary for Safer Drug Use

- Try to make significant lifestyle changes that may allow you to avoid taking the medication in the first place. Even if your physician has started you on a medication, effective lifestyle changes may allow your particular problem to improve enough that your physician could possibly discontinue its use in the future. (See Chapter 14.)
- Make a list of all prescription medications, over-the-counter drugs, herbal therapies, and nutritional supplements you are taking, and put them on a card that will fit in your billfold or purse so that you will always have it available.
- Discuss the potential side effects and adverse drug reactions of any new drug that your physician has prescribed with him and with your pharmacist.

- Ask if this medication will interact with any of the medications you are presently taking.
- Discuss the desired therapeutic goals your doctor has with this new medication.
- Choose drugs that have been on the market for at least five years.
- Read all the directions, precautions, and potential adverse reactions that should accompany any new script the pharmacist fills.
- Become established with a primary-care physician who is willing to coordinate all of your care and medications.
- Seek out additional information from books, the *Physicians' Desk Reference*, or the Internet. (See the resource section in the addendum of this book.)
- Follow carefully all recommendations for future lab work and checkups with your physician.
- Be sure that the drug you are taking actually meets the goals you originally established with your physician. If it doesn't, be sure to ask if you can discontinue it and try a different medication or therapy.
- Most important rule: If you feel that you could be reacting in any way to your medication, contact your primary-care physician immediately. Discontinue the use of the drug, if possible, until this question is totally resolved.

We will forever be vulnerable to the choices of others. Institutions and governmental agencies continue to make decisions that are out of our control. But we have more influence than we often realize. I hope I've empowered you to make safe and effective choices with prescription medicine in the future.

———

Groundskeepers are safe and effective, yet it took only one innocent oversight to cut a power line that triggered an entire chain of events that will literally take weeks to fix. Will I give up on groundskeepers and never trust another one? That would be silly. Even though they use dangerous tools, I need them. Their benefits far outweigh the risks involved. You can bet, however, that I'll not hesitate to question the next one if he's digging next to the power box on my lawn!

The same is true for prescription drugs. They can be safe and effective *within reason*, but we must be intentional and sometimes even aggressive in seeking additional information. Listen to your body and ask as many questions as necessary. I don't know much about planting trees, and I can pretty much guarantee that when I question a professional, he will give me a little attitude. I think it's worth the gamble, don't you?

CHAPTER FOURTEEN

Health Concepts

WHILE CONDUCTING THE RESEARCH FOR THIS BOOK, I'VE become more and more overwhelmed by the staggering dependence our society and medical community places on prescription medication, over-the-counter drugs, and herbs. Few of us seriously consider the poor lifestyle habits that may be the underlying cause of the problem.

Excessive weight may account for painful knees, aching hips, high blood pressure, diabetes, increases in acid reflux symptoms, and fatigue. Smoking causes increased risks in high blood pressure, heart disease, emphysema, and lung cancer. Poor eating habits contribute to high cholesterol, high blood pressure, and diabetes. Lack of physical activity can lead to osteoporosis, obesity, diabetes, high blood pressure, decreased immune function, and high stress levels. When people go to their physicians' offices for help after developing these problems, almost invariably their doctors place them on medication while paying little attention to the underlying lifestyles that are most likely the main culprit.

Dr. Mark Nelson reported in the *American Journal of Hypertension* that 42 percent of patients with hypertension could get off their medication if they would follow simple lifestyle changes.[1] The Diabetes Prevention Study showed that even patients with glucose intolerance could avoid becoming diabetic over 50 percent of the time by simply adopting a moderate exercise program and improving their eating habits.[2] The medical literature strongly supports a trial of healthy lifestyle changes for patients who have developed high blood pressure, diabetes, or elevated cholesterol prior to starting any medication.

Physicians most often lack the time or desire to inform patients specifically of what they need to do to be proactive about their health. Even when doctors do comment about lifestyle changes, they typically do so while writing the patient a prescription, assuming he will not make the necessary changes. They prescribe medication as the only hope of improving patients' health, and we have accepted this as a reasonable response.

Traditional Preventive Medicine

A resigned attitude has crept over our nation. People today are living shorter and dying longer. The overwhelming majority of Americans today expect that they, too, will develop one or several chronic degenerative diseases. When they do, they will try to catch it early and turn to modern medicine as their savior.

The health-care community likes to pride itself in the fact that it promotes preventive care. Physicians encourage patients to have routine physicals in order to maintain health. Yet a closer look quickly leads one to the conclusion that physicians are primarily trying to detect disease earlier.

> People today are living shorter and dying longer.

Pap smears, PSAs (Prostate Specific Antigen— a screening test for prostate cancer), mammograms, blood work, and physical exams are merely attempts to find a silent disease the patient may already have. Obviously, the earlier you detect disease, the better it is for you, but then you still haven't prevented anything. Physicians spend very little time or effort teaching patients effective lifestyle changes that could allow them to avoid getting these illnesses in the first place.

Attitudes are changing, however. I believe the pendulum is swinging toward a more proactive approach to improving one's lifestyle with less reliance on medication. As the baby-boomer generation begins to turn fifty, more and more individuals are aggressively looking for better solutions. By combining the best that traditional medicine has to offer and incorporating healthy lifestyles, everyone has the best chance of protecting his health.

> By combining the best that traditional medicine has to offer and incorporating healthy lifestyles, everyone has the best chance of protecting his health.

With just a little encouragement, approximately 80 percent of my patients choose to make healthy lifestyle changes that improve their underlying medical conditions. Granted, I have patients who will not consider making *any* changes, and for them I have no other alternative than to write prescriptions.

Healthy Lifestyle Changes As a First Choice—Medications As a Last Resort

There is tremendous ambiguity in the area of wellness and preventive medicine today. Every individual who makes a decision to choose a healthier lifestyle will find plenty of conflicting information. We are bombarded with magazine articles, talk shows, demonstrations, flyers, and best-selling books, each proclaiming previously unknown secrets and "cutting-edge" health information. The Internet offers endless resources, both good and bad. Where should you turn?

Families want a personal connection and look to their physicians as the authority on health-care issues that stretch beyond the topic of disease. They're asking for guidance on diet, exercise, supplements, and herbal therapies. How disappointing it is to find that even though every physician understands that eating habits and lack of exercise are at the core of many diseases, most remain strictly disease- and drug-oriented and usually discourage their patients' use of any complementary medicine. The American public has long displayed an avid interest in the relations of diet and health, and our expectations for guidelines on nutrition and exercise are becoming more and more sophisticated. Still, the authority patients most wish to consult for guidance remains insufficiently informed about the role of diet, exercise, and nutritional supplementation in the prevention and treatment of disease.

Now that you realize the inherent risk you and your family assume by taking any medication (even over-the-counter medication and herbs), you too may be thinking, *I need to protect my health.* The absolute best way of avoiding a serious adverse drug reaction is to not need any medication in the first place. The human body God created is amazing in its ability to heal. Our bodies are truly marvelously and wonderfully made.

> The absolute best way of avoiding a serious adverse drug reaction is to not need any medication in the first place.

The most important principle I have learned over the past seven years of research is that the body's natural immune system, natural repair system, and natural antioxidant defense system, which the Great Physician designed, are the best means of protecting one's health—not the drugs I can prescribe.

In the rest of this chapter I will briefly summarize a healthy lifestyle. During the past several years, I have specialized in nutritional medicine. I have researched literally thousands of medical studies that have appeared in our mainline medical journals, which focused on how a healthy diet, modest exercise program, and nutritional supplementation can protect our health. This triad of healthy lifestyle habits is the absolute best way for you to avoid an adverse drug reaction. If you can prevent these chronic degenerative diseases from occurring in the first place, your doctor won't need to start his medication in the first place. By following these simple guidelines, you, too, can take charge of maintaining your health.

Enjoy the life God has given you while being a good steward in providing for and protecting your body. This choice requires motivation and commitment, but unlike the dilemma with prescription medicine, the benefits far outweigh the risk.

Basic Healthy Diet

What we eat has an enormous effect on our overall health. Thousands of studies support the idea that diet is highly correlated with the risk of

> ### Benefits of a Healthy Diet
>
> - Weight loss
> - Decreased risk of diabetes
> - Decreased risk of heart disease
> - Decreased risk of almost all cancers
> - Decreased risk of high blood pressure
> - Lower cholesterol levels
> - Enhanced immune system
> - Increased sensitivity to insulin
> - Increased energy and ability to concentrate

developing various chronic degenerative diseases. Food is, in fact, our greatest drug. We can use it either incorrectly and cause great problems or correctly and protect our health.

Recent studies have shown that by eating a healthy diet and exercising moderately, we can significantly reduce the risk of developing diabetes, heart disease, cancer, and a host of other chronic degenerative diseases. The diet I recommend takes into consideration many of these potential medical problems. I am not a nutritionist; it is rather from a doctor's point of view that I lay the foundation for a balanced diet.

Carbohydrates

Carbohydrates are simply long chains of sugars that are released and absorbed at various rates in our bodies. They include fruits, vegetables, grains, and sugars. The medical community believes that the more simple the sugar (for example, table sugar, candy, or soda pop) one consumes, the faster the sugar is absorbed into the bloodstream and the quicker one's blood sugar rises. A new concept is now being studied, which is called the glycemic index. The glycemic index—or how fast our bodies absorb a particular carbohydrate—is determined by studying each individual carbohydrate. Few of us realize that highly processed carbohydrates such as white bread, white flour, rice, and potatoes actually release their sugars faster than table sugar. These foods are considered *high-glycemic carbohydrates*.[3]

On the other hand, carbohydrates such as cauliflower, beans, asparagus, apples, oranges, and grapes release their sugars more slowly, thus keeping blood sugars from spiking. These carbohydrates are called *low-glycemic*. Furthermore, these carbs contain high amounts of fiber—the indigestible portion of our food. Fiber passes through the gastrointestinal tract without being absorbed, not only allowing our nutrients to be absorbed at a much slower pace, but also helping to eliminate toxins as it cleanses the colon. An increased amount of fiber is very important in our overall diet and can be found in fruits, vegetables, and whole grains.[4]

I recommend between thirty-five and fifty grams of fiber each day. Most Americans consume only eight to ten grams of fiber per day and have come to believe that a bowel movement every other day is more than sufficient. Our paradigm is limited. Perhaps a broader worldview would prove enlightening.

The late Dr. Denis Burkitt, a Christian surgeon famous for discovering the disease *Burkitt's lymphoma,* practiced medicine in Africa for more than twenty years. While there, he hardly saw a single case of colon cancer, diverticulitis, hemorrhoids, gall-bladder disease, or even appendicitis in the native population. He attributed this remarkable finding to the fact that his native African patients consumed sixty to seventy grams of fiber per day and typically had three to five bowel movements every day. When Dr. Burkitt returned to the United States in the late 1970s, he spent most of his time promoting the health benefits of a high-fiber diet.

Constipation is a $3 billion business in the United States alone. When I refer a patient to the gastroenterologist, I can count on the fact is that he will recommend that my patient eat more fiber. The fiber in low-glycemic carbohydrates provides most of this necessary substance. However, many of us need to supplement our diet with additional fiber in order to obtain the thirty-five to fifty grams needed each day. I guarantee the tremendous health benefits you will reap by making this intentional effort will prove worthwhile.

Glucose (the basic sugar the body uses; the one to which all carbohydrates eventually break down) is extremely easy for the body to absorb and in turn raises blood sugar rapidly. The rate at which the blood sugar increases (the glycemic index) is rated at one hundred. In contrast, fructose (found in fruits) is more difficult for the body to absorb and is therefore considered low-glycemic, with an index of nineteen.

> Rice cakes, one of our favorite diet foods, have one of the highest glycemic indexes of any food.

White table sugar has a glycemic index of sixty-five because it is a disaccharide (made up of two molecules: one molecule of glucose and one molecule of fructose).

Surprising to many, wheat and white bread actually have a very high glycemic index (even higher than that of table sugar) because of their physical structure. The fine particle size and the exploded structure the leavening action of the yeast causes makes the surface of wheat starch extremely accessible to digestive enzymes. These foods are actually worse for our bodies than table sugar because of how quickly their absorption raises blood sugar. Rice cakes, one of our favorite diet foods, have one of the highest glycemic indexes of any food.[5]

The average dietitian does not utilize the glycemic index, which was introduced in the early 1980s. A recent study in the *Journal of American Medical Association,* however, points out the potential serious outcome of consuming great quantities of high-glycemic foods in America and most industrialized nations. Problems such as hypertension, obesity, elevated cholesterol and triglycerides, heart attacks, strokes, and diabetes are primarily related to our diet.[6]

Dr. Walter Willet, head of nutrition and preventive medicine at Harvard, says in his book *Eat, Drink, and Be Healthy* (Simon and Schuster, 2001) that white bread, white flours, rice, and potatoes should be placed at the top of the food pyramid with sweets and snacks. In turn, I encourage my patients to eat less bread (or to choose heavy multigrain brands) and more carbohydrates high in fiber.

We need to balance low-glycemic carbohydrates with good proteins and good fats. When in a meal we combine good protein and good fat with low-glycemic carbohydrates, we slow the absorption of sugar and stimulate the release of glucagon (the hormone opposite of insulin). This actually reverses all of the bad metabolic changes that occur with elevated blood levels of insulin (high blood pressure, elevated triglycerides, lower HDL cholesterol, central obesity).

Good Proteins

Protein has been maligned over the years due to the tremendous focus on low-fat diets. Since proteins contain most of the "bad" fats, we have thrown the protein out with the fat. People have been led to believe that a high-carbohydrate, low-fat diet is the healthiest diet we can eat. Yet the amino acids found only in proteins are essential for all of our body's functions, especially our immune system. We must choose good protein sources.

Vegetable proteins are the very best ones we can eat, their greatest advantage being that they contain fewer environmental toxins and chemicals than animal protein. Vegetable proteins also contain the good fat and provide the highly needed antioxidants we all need. Some good sources of plant protein are soy, legumes, beans, and nuts. By consuming a wide variety of plant foods, you are able to provide your body with all the essential proteins while also providing much-needed good fat.

Cold-water fish offers the next best source of protein. Salmon, mackerel, sardines, and tuna not only give you a good source of protein but also much-needed sources of omega-3 essential fatty acids, which I will discuss more under fats. Again, be aware of toxins these fish may contain due to industrial pollution of our waters. Mercury poisoning as well as many other toxins are increasing in all fish species. Shellfish and larger saltwater fish are the worst. Knowing the source of the fish is helpful.

Fowl are the next best source of protein. Chicken and turkey are most favorable because the fat accumulates on the outside of the meat rather than on the inside. Since most toxins found in these animals accumulate in the fat, you can easily avoid them by removing the skin and fat from the meat. Organically grown fowl is a great choice if it is available to you.

Animal products are less desirable sources of protein due to high levels of saturated fat marbled inside red meat. I encourage my patients to keep their consumption of red meat to a minimum. Knowing that many like to have a good steak once in a while, I recommend that those patients choose the leanest cut they can get. Remember, *no one* needs to consume the twenty-four-ounce cut. Eat small, fine cuts of steak along with tasty low-glycemic vegetables. You do need to avoid such meats as bacon, hot dogs, salami, and lunch meats. You should also skip organ meats (liver, brain, and kidney) due to high toxin concentrations.

Dairy products are the least desirable protein source because they have the highest concentration of saturated fats. Milk, eggs, cheese, butter, and buttermilk rank among some of the unhealthiest foods. Few people are willing to eliminate dairy products because they make our recipes taste so good, but you can markedly improve your diet by eating low-fat or nonfat milk and cheese. If you eat eggs, consider eating more egg whites than egg yolks. Range-fed chickens produce eggs that contain helpful omega-3 fatty acids. We will all be much healthier if we keep the total amount of saturated fats to a minimum.

Good Fats

Proteins have been given a bad rap, but not nearly to the degree of fats. The consumption of fats in our diet has certainly been the talk of this past half-century. Still, people are as confused about fats today as they were a generation ago. In fact, in many ways they are even more confused. The bottom line is: our bodies need fats to thrive. Many aspects of the cell, but especially the formation of the cell membrane, require fat. Our bodies use fat also for the production of many of our hormones, natural anti-inflammatories, and basic energy needs. Not only must we discern between good and bad fats, but we need to know how and when to consume what kind of fats for good health.

The bottom line is: our bodies need fats to thrive.

Saturated fats. These come primarily from animal fat and dairy products. These are the worst fats that we can consume. Saturated fats increase total cholesterol and LDL, or "bad" cholesterol, and lower HDL, or "good" cholesterol. Most Americans and people of industrialized nations consume the majority of their fats in the form of saturated fats. Numerous studies reveal that the actual consumption of cholesterol does little to increase our cholesterol levels; however, the consumption of saturated fats and high-glycemic carbohydrates plays a large part in elevating cholesterol and triglyceride levels. Most nutritionists now realize that it is not simply the fat in our diet causing problems, but rather the types of fats we are consuming.

Polyunsaturated fats. In the 1950s, polyunsaturated fats became popular as a "healthy" substitute for saturated fats. For example, vegetable oils were made into margarine as a substitute for butter. Vegetable oils primarily contain what is known as polyunsaturated fats. These fats do in fact lower LDL, or "bad" cholesterol, but the problem is that they also lower HDL, or "good" cholesterol. Polyunsaturated fats are also vulnerable to oxidation and easily transform into *trans-fatty acids,* which are rancid fats. These fats make poor building blocks for our cell membranes and are anything but healthy.

Many vegetable oils now go through a process called *partial hydrogenation.* The reason food manufacturers go to the trouble of this process is to improve taste, spreadability, pleasurable sensation in the mouth, and to extend shelf life. It has nothing to do with making a "healthy" alternative.

To hydrogenate oils, manufacturers heat the oils to high temperatures under pressure with hydrogen gas, but the process is stopped before it is completed. This abbreviated process provides a mixture of both saturated and polyunsaturated fats, with a high concentration of trans-fatty acids. When you look at food labels you will be amazed how many processed foods are made of partially hydrogenated fats. I recommend avoiding these kinds of fats altogether.

Monosaturated fats. We consider these healthy fats because they actually help lower LDL cholesterol while maintaining HDL cholesterol levels. We find them in such foods as cashews, avocados, olive oil, and pistachio nuts. Virgin olive oil is a very good source of monosaturated fats; so are canola and peanut oils. Even though these fats do not contain the essential fatty acids, they appear to be much healthier and in some ways protective against heart disease.[7]

Essential fats: omega-3 and omega-6 essential fatty acids. These essential fats are just that—essential. They fall into the category of polyunsaturated fats and are very good fats when they are not highly processed or heated. Our bodies cannot make them, so we need to get them from our diet. We get plenty of omega-6 fatty acids in the Western diet; however, almost all of us are deficient in the omega-3 fatty acids.

Omega-6 fatty acids produce hormones (*prostaglandins*) that promote inflammation, cell growth, and blood clotting. Omega-3 fatty acids produce prostaglandins with just the opposite effect. In the event that you are injured, you need to have a good inflammatory response to bring about quicker healing—the inflammatory response brings blood and immune cells to the wounded area. But if you have not been hurt, an inflammatory response can damage tissue and cause major problems—for example, asthma, arthritis, and heart disease. Therefore it is critical that we consume these essential fats in a balanced fashion so that the hormones they produce will also occur in balance. Unbalanced prostaglandins can cause serious health problems such as cancer, heart disease, inflammatory diseases, and autoimmune diseases.

Omega-6 fatty acids are found in meats, margarines, peanuts, poultry, and many of our processed foods. Omega-3 fatty acids are found in cold-water fish, flaxseed, soybeans, organic eggs, almonds, and oils made from flaxseed. It is most beneficial to consume these essential fats in a ratio of two omega-6 fatty acids to one omega-3 fatty acid (2:1 ratio). But Americans consume an estimated ratio of 20:1, and in some cases 40:1. Is it any wonder we are in a health crisis?

It is imperative that you make a concerted effort to consume foods high in omega-3 fatty acids in order to balance out these two essential fats. Eating adequate quantities of the omega-3 fatty acids will actually lower your total cholesterol and LDL cholesterol. Most people simply need to supplement their diet with cold-pressed flaxseed, sunflower, pumpkin-seed oils, or fish oil. Or better yet—they should replace most of the saturated fat with these fats.

I realize most people will eat saturated fats and, at times, even partially hydrogenated fats. Still, it is important to get the majority of your fats from essential fatty acids and monosaturated fats.

Combining Carbohydrates, Proteins, and Fats

It is critical that you have a portion of carbohydrates, proteins, and fats with each meal or snack. Every time we eat, we need balanced nutrition, making certain not to spike our blood sugars. Learn to eat for hormonal control rather than caloric control. Insulin is our "storage" hormone and most of us do not want to put on any more fat than we already have. Glucagon, the fat-burning hormone, actually takes fat and utilizes it as an energy source. It is critical that when you eat a meal or snack you do not overstimulate the release of insulin. This can lead to insulin resistance (you are simply not as sensitive to your insulin as you once were), which can lead to heart disease, stroke, diabetes, and obesity. This is why it is imperative to eat a well-balanced diet, which is made up of good protein, good fat, and good carbohydrates. I explain to my patients who are overweight that by eating a balance of carbohydrates, proteins, and fats, the side effect is fat loss. If you don't need to lose any weight, then you won't. You will feel less hungry and more energetic.

I believe that approximately 40 to 50 percent of our calories should come from low-glycemic carbohydrates, 25 to 30 percent of our calories from good proteins, and 25 to 30 percent of our calories from good fats. Several different ratios will accomplish this same overall goal. In his book *The Zone*, Barry Sears recommends the 40/30/30 ratio—40 percent carbohydrates, 30 percent protein, and 30 percent fat. Other diets recommend 50 percent carbohydrates, 30 percent protein, and 20 percent fat. The goal is to accomplish stable hormonal results, which are necessary for a healthy lifestyle.

Here are some principles to help you get started:

- Be careful not to take in too many high-glycemic carbohydrates with any particular meal, especially when eating out. Don't eat bread, potatoes, and dessert all at the same meal.
- Be creative with your snacks and be sure that they contain the right balance of carbs, good fats, and good proteins.
- Always have healthy snacks readily available. If you don't, you will eat whatever is around when you get hungry.
- Purchase lean nutrition bars (I like Balance bars) and lean drinks, which already have the proper balance, and keep them readily available.
- You will tend to have some withdrawal from a high-carbohydrate diet. But once you become consistent with this diet you will feel much better, with a marked increase in energy.

Most people find it relatively easy to stay with eating this way because it is simply a health diet and can easily become part of your lifestyle. Be creative using these principles and enjoy your food. Please refer to the Resource Section at the end of this book for references on eating a healthy diet.

Healthy Exercise Program

Benefits of a Modest Exercise Program

- Weight loss
- Lower blood pressure
- Builds stronger bones and decreases the risk of osteoporosis
- Elevates the HDL "good" cholesterol
- Lowers total cholesterol and LDL "bad" cholesterol
- Improves sensitivity to insulin, which decreases triglyceride levels
- Enhances the immune system
- Increases strength and coordination, which leads to decreased risk of falls
- Overall increases one's sense of well-being[8]

Everyone knows that moderate, consistent exercise is essential to a healthy lifestyle. The body was designed to be active. Isn't it amazing how the human body has the capacity to withstand natural calamity, cross barren deserts, and scale sheer, icy cliffs? History has proven the body's incredible ability of strength and endurance. The one condition a body cannot survive, however, is inactivity.

The challenge for many of us with desk jobs or for those who are elderly is to know how best to utilize our limited time for the most beneficial results. Exercise gurus continually debate the best type and duration of exercise, but as a physician, I have a different attitude about how one should approach developing an exercise program. My primary concern is not appearance or fast results. I am concerned about health and longevity. It is more important to exercise consistently than to worry about how to exercise. Any exercise program is better than none. For those who are serious about increasing or maintaining their well-being, I suggest the following:

- Choose an exercise program in which you can remain consistent. You need to enjoy the exercise program as much as possible so you will stay with it.
- Schedule workouts instead of trying to work an exercise program into your existing schedule. I can testify that this does not work— my schedule always wins out.
- Don't overdo it. Be careful not to injure yourself when starting an exercise program. Most of us have not been in good shape for years, if ever.
- Start slowly, and gradually increase the length and intensity of your workouts. It is not a race. Your strength and endurance will increase.
- For those with any joint or musculoskeletal problems, I recommend seeing a physical therapist who can guide an exercise program and help prevent injury.
- For those with any risk of coronary artery disease or who are more than forty years old, I recommend first seeing a physician

and obtaining an exercise stress test from a cardiologist before embarking on any exercise program.

A simple walking program offers numerous health benefits. If my patients want to swim, ride a bike, play racquetball, basketball, or even walk while golfing, I encourage them to do so. I have found, however, that a combination of aerobics with strength training is the ideal workout program.

Benefits of Strength/Resistance Training

We've all heard the benefits of aerobic exercise over the last several decades. But many people still react negatively to the idea of strength or resistance training, thinking of bodybuilding or training as just for athletes. Yet strength or resistance training offers positive fitness and health benefits for ordinary adults of all ages.

In a well-designed program, resistance training can provide increased challenge to the long bones of the upper extremities, the spine, pelvis, and ribs. This can produce positive results for those who may have, or who are prone to have, osteoporosis. Generally an aerobics program will stress only the lower extremities.

When losing weight, many are not concerned whether they drop muscle mass along with the fat mass; they just want to "lose weight." Resistance training can prevent the loss of muscle mass while aiding in your fat-loss effort. Since muscle is the furnace that burns the body's fuel, glucose, the more muscle mass you have, the easier it is to maintain your optimal body weight.

> Exercise, including strength training, helps to make the body more sensitive to its natural insulin not only during, but following exercise sessions.

Aerobic exercise helps to make the body more sensitive to its natural insulin not only during, but following exercise sessions. This is a great benefit to those who have diabetes mellitus or for those who want to avoid becoming diabetic.

It was once believed that the loss of muscle mass, especially in the upper body, was a normal part of the aging process. This is far from the truth. Strength training not only helps prevent the loss of muscle mass associated with aging but can actually increase muscle mass even for those in their eighties and nineties. It is a known fact that we begin losing muscle mass after age thirty-five unless we are involved in strength training.

Studies also indicate that healthy, elderly individuals who are stronger are less likely to have frequent falls. An appropriately designed resistance program can also help maintain flexibility and balance. You can enhance these benefits by adding stretch exercises. A well-designed workout can also have significant cardiovascular benefits. Resistance training plays a vital role in preventing heart attacks by conditioning the cardiovascular system to cope more efficiently with sudden changes in blood pressure and heart rate.

Strive for a balance of aerobics, resistance training, and stretching in your exercise program. I recommend modest aerobics at least three times a week and strength training twice a week.

Rest is also an essential aspect to health. Did you know our bodies actually become stronger during rest? You should allow your body a break of at least two days each week.

Nutritional Supplementation

The final aspect of a healthy lifestyle is nutritional supplementation. For years I told my patients they could get everything their bodies needed from their diets. After researching the medical literature for the past eight years on the subject, however, I am convinced that every man, woman, and child needs to be taking nutritional supplements. Why?

Medical literature has shown oxidative stress (the dark side of oxygen) to be the underlying cause of more than seventy chronic degenerative diseases such as heart disease, cancer, stroke, macular degeneration, arthritis, and Alzheimer's dementia. Remember, oxidative stress is created by excessive charged oxygen molecules, called free radicals. In fact, many researchers now believe that oxidative stress is one of the leading causes of the aging process itself.[9]

It is impossible to cover this subject effectively in a few paragraphs. In fact, I have written an entire book devoted to what I believe is the most important aspect of protecting your health—nutritional supplementation. *What Your Doctor Doesn't Know About Nutritional Medicine May Be Killing You* explains that most physicians are not aware of how oxidative stress can destroy our health and how nutritional supplements are our best defense against the damage it can cause. I based this book on scientific literature and present the medical evidence that demands a verdict. Should you be taking nutritional supplements?

Building up your body's natural antioxidant defense system, natural repair system, and natural immune system through supplementation is critical in maintaining your health. Our bodies have complicated and sophisticated antioxidant defense systems to protect us from the devastating damage of oxidative stress. Because our generation is under greater attack from the toxins in our environment, our stressful lifestyles, and poor eating habits than any other previous generation, we need to optimize these defense systems. Eating a healthy diet is a good a start. But there is no way we can obtain the optimal levels of the nutrients our bodies need from our diets alone. We must supplement our diets to best protect our health.

Health Benefits of Nutritional Supplements

- Enhance the immune system
- Enhance the antioxidant defense system
- Decrease the risk of heart attacks, strokes, and cancer
- Decrease the risk of arthritis, macular degeneration, and cataracts
- Decrease the risk of asthma and hay fever
- Decrease the risk of Alzheimer's dementia, Parkinson's disease, and many other chronic degenerative diseases

---

Physicians are usually negative about their patients taking any kind of supplements. But once you understand that oxidative stress is the root cause of almost all of our major chronic degenerative diseases, you will agree that supplementing your healthy diet with high-quality supplements is essential.

I recommend taking an antioxidant tablet and a mineral tablet containing a wide variety of antioxidants at optimal levels. These nutrients work synergistically. I call this *cellular nutrition*. Cellular nutrition is simply providing all the nutrients to the cell at optimal levels—not at RDA (Recommended Daily Allowance) levels—allowing the cell to decide what it does and does not need. See my Resource Page for some recommended supplements.

Optimal levels are those levels of supplementation that research has shown to provide a health benefit. The problem is not one of nutritional deficiency, but instead of oxidative stress. I would encourage you to read my book to fully understand these concepts of supplementation. In the meantime, Table 1 will give you a basic guideline of what I would consider optimal levels and the variety needed in your supplements to offer cellular nutrition.

Table 1

Basic Nutritional Supplement Recommendations	
ANTIOXIDANTS	The more and varied your antioxidants, the better.
VITAMIN A	I do not recommend the use of straight vitamin A because of its potential toxicity. Instead supplement with a mixture of mixed carotenoids. Carotenoids become vitamin A in the body as the body has need and they have no toxicity problems.
CAROTENOIDS	It is important to have a mixture of carotenoids rather than taking only beta-carotene. • Beta-carotene—10,000 to 15,000 IU • Lycopene—1 to 3 mg • Lutein/Zeaxanthin—1 to 6 mg • Alpha carotene—500 to 800 mcg
VITAMIN C	A mixture of vitamin C is important, especially calcium, potassium, zinc, and magnesium ascorbates, which are much more potent in handling oxidative stress. • 1000 to 2000 mg

Table 1, continued

VITAMIN E	It is important to be getting a mixture of natural vitamin Es: d-alpha tocopherol, d-gamma tocopherol, and mixed tocotrienol. • 400 to 800 IU
BIOFLAVANOID COMPLEX OF ANTIOXIDANTS	Bioflavanoids offer a necessary variety of potent antioxidants and are a great asset to your supplements. The amounts may vary but should include the majority of the following: • Rutin • Quercetin • Broccoli • Green Tea • Cruciferous • Bilberry • Grape-Seed Extract • Bromelain
ALPHA-LIPOIC ACID	• 15 to 30 mg
CoQ10	• 20 to 30 mg
GLUTATHIONE	• 10 to 20 mg • Precursor: N-acetyl-L-cysteine—50 to 75 mg
B VITAMINS (COFACTORS)	• Folic Acid—800 to 1000 mcg • Vitamin B1 (Thiamin)—20 to 30 mg • Vitamin B2 (Riboflavin)—25 to 50 mg • Vitamin B3 (Niacin)—30 to 75 mg • Vitamin B5 (Pantothenic Acid)—80 to 200 mg • Vitamin B6 (Pyridoxine)—25 to 50 mg • Vitamin B12 (Cobalamin)—100 to 250 mcg • Biotin—300 to 1,000 mcg
OTHER IMPORTANT VITAMINS	• Vitamin D3 (Cholecalciferol)—450 IU to 800 IU • Vitamin K—50 to 100 mcg
MINERAL COMPLEX	• Calcium—800 to 1,500 mg depending on your dietary intake of calcium • Magnesium—500 to 800 mg • Zinc—20 to 30 mg • Selenium—200 mcg is ideal • Chromium—200 to 300 mcg • Copper—1 to 3 mg • Manganese—3 to 6 mg • Vanadium—30 to 100 mcg • Iodine—100 to 200 mcg • Molybdenum—50 to 100 mcg • Mixture of Trace Minerals
ADDITIONAL NUTRIENTS FOR BONE HEALTH	• Silicon—3 mg • Boron—2 to 3 mg

Table 1, continued

OTHER IMPORTANT AND ESSENTIAL NUTRIENTS Improved Homocysteine levels and improved brain function	• Choline----100 to 200 mg • Trimethylglycine----200 to 500 mg • Inositol----150mg to 250 mg

Supplementing Your Diet

ESSENTIAL FATS:	• Cold-Pressed Flaxseed oil • Fish Oil Capsules
FIBER SUPPLEMENT	• Blend of soluble and insoluble fiber----10 to 30 mg depending on your dietary consumption of fiber (ideal is 35 to 50 grams of total fiber daily)

** *Several nutritional companies are putting together these essential nutrients into one or two different tablets, which need to be taken 2 to 3 times daily in order to achieve this level of supplementation. Look for a high-quality product that comes as close as possible to these recommendations. If the manufacturer follows pharmaceutical GMP and USP guidelines, you will be giving yourself the absolute best protection against oxidative stress.* **See the Resource Page for some suggested supplements.**

The essential fats and fiber provide added nutrients that are usually missing in the Western diet.

Since the supplementation industry is essentially an unregulated market, I recommend taking a high-quality supplement that is manufactured by a company that follows Good Manufacturing Practices (GMP) as a pharmaceutical. This means it makes its supplements much like a drug company that is producing an over-the-counter medication. It is also important that these tablets dissolve. Be sure to consume supplements that also follow USP guidelines for the dissolution of the tablet. Please see the Appendix pages at the end of this book for help in discerning whether or not your supplements meet the USP guidelines. It also includes information on a few companies that I am familiar with that follow GMP.

It is much easier and safer to maintain your health than to try to regain it once you've lost it. A healthy, proactive lifestyle is always your best protection against suffering an adverse drug reaction. It is impossible to suffer from a drug reaction when you don't need drugs, right?

———————

I realize that most of us will take medication (or several medications) during our lifetimes; thus, my purpose in writing this book is to help you avoid the potential dangers inherent within every medication on the market today. Please know that you have not heard me advise you to stop seeing doctors or to throw away all prescription meds. Though

> It is much easier and safer to maintain your health than to try to regain it once you've lost it.

suffering and/or dying from an adverse drug reaction remains an undeniably high risk for our nation, without a doubt we can avoid it without extreme reactions to the medical community.

It is our blind faith that I address here. Blind faith in pharmaceutical companies, the FDA, physicians, or pharmacists is not acceptable when medications are known to be the third leading cause of death in this country!

While researching and writing this book, I found that one simple truth encouraged me to challenge the establishment and shine a light onto the *true dangers of prescription medication*: the medical literature states over and over again that more than half of these injuries and deaths can and should be prevented. And yet I did not find evidence of anyone doing anything about it.

Are you one of the 50 percent whose injury or death can be avoided? Who will make certain that you don't become a statistic? By following the basic guidelines and precautions presented here, *you* will decrease your risk of suffering or dying from an adverse drug reaction. Above all, never forget that *you* are the most important player in this chain of events.

Be informed. Be proactive. Be bold.

May it never be said that yours was a death by prescription.

Appendix: Resources

LEARNING MORE ABOUT EACH DRUG YOU OR YOUR LOVED ones take is critical for safety. There are several books available that can teach you about your particular medications. I recommend that you browse through some of these reference books at your local bookstore, and decide which one seems easiest to use and most understandable. If you are taking several medications, you may also want to invest in a book on drug interactions. Also listed below is information on a few companies that produce nutritional products using Good Manufacturing Practices, which I discuss in Chapter 14.

Resource Books for Pharmaceutical Drugs:

1. Graedon, Joe, and Teresa Graedon, Ph.D. *The People's Guide to Deadly Drug Interactions.* New York: St. Martin's Press, 1997.
2. *Physicians' Desk Reference.* Montvale, N.J.: Medical Economics Company, 2003.
3. Rybacki, James, Pharm.D., and James Long, M.D. *The Essential Guide to Prescription Drugs 2001.* New York: Harper Collins, 2002.
4. Silverman, Harold, Pharm.D. *The Pill Book—Guide to Safe Drug Use.* New York: Bantam, 1989.
5. Tatro, David. *Drug Interaction Facts.* St. Louis, Mo.: Facts and Comparisons, 2003.
6. Wolfe, Sidney, M.D., Larry Sasich, Pharm.D., and Rose-Ellen Hope, R.Ph. *Worst Pills—Best Pills.* New York: Pocket Books Health, 1999.

Resource Books for Herbal Drugs:

1. Ringer, David, ed., *Physicians' Guide to Nutriceuticals.* Omaha, Nebr.: Nutritional Data Resources, 1998.
2. Werbach, Melvyn, M.D., and Michael Murray, N.D. *Botanical Influences on Illness.* New York: Third Line Press, 1994.

Resources for Nutritional Supplements:

1. Strand, Ray D., M.D. *What Your Doctor Doesn't Know About Nutritional Medicine May Be Killing You.* Nashville, Tenn.: Thomas Nelson, 2002.

Below are some sources for nutritional supplements that provide cellular nutrition and follow USP and pharmaceutical-GMP (Good Manufacturing Practices). This is obviously not a complete list; however, these are few with which I am familiar:

1. Usana Essentials*—Mega Antioxidant and Chelated Mineral. Manufactured by Usana Health Sciences, Inc. You need to take three of each daily, preferably one antioxidant and one mineral tablet with each meal. To order, call 888-950-9595. For more information, log on to their Web site at www.usana.com.
2. Multigenics Intensive Care Formula without Iron. Manufactured by Metagenics. You need to take eight tablets daily. These are only available through health-care providers. Log on to www.metagenics.com to find a health-care professional close to you.
3. Life Extension Mix Tabs, Mix Caps, or Mix Powder. Manufactured by Life Extension Foundation. You need to take either 9 tablets, 14 capsules, or three scoops of powder daily. To order, call 800-544-4440 or log on to www.LifeExtension.com.
4. Supra Vita-CoQ10 Formula Caplets (Iron-Free). Manufactured by Bluebonnet Nutrition Corporation. You need to take 3 daily (does not provide the optimal level of all the nutrients recommended; however, it is still a good formula). You can purchase this at your local health-food store.

* These are the products I am personally recommending to my patients.

Internet Resources for Pharmaceutical Drugs:

The one big disadvantage of purchasing books for drug information is the fact that most of them are outdated before they are even released. New drugs are being released monthly, new adverse drug reactions are being discovered daily, and new drug interactions are being realized as the Post-Marketing Surveillance program is slowly working. Therefore, I recommend that patients who have access to the Internet and are comfortable using it search for sites that can give them more information about the particular drugs they are taking. Realize that there is always good information and bad information found throughout the Internet. The best site I have located to give you good, credible information about your drugs and drug interactions is found at *www.drugstore.com.*

1. Click on the Pharmacy tab on the home page.
2. Click on drug prices on the pharmacy page.
   a. Enter the name of the drug in which you are interested, and click on "Go."
   b. Scroll down the page to find information on the drug and frequently asked questions about it.
3. When you are on the pharmacy page you can also click on "Drug Interaction Checker."
   a. Begin entering the name of each drug you are taking, one at a time.
   b. Be sure to also enter any vitamins, herbs, or over-the-counter medications.
   c. Once you have entered the names of all your medications, click on the "Go" tab.
   d. Then print this information for your review and for your records.
4. Also located on this site is the option for an "eMedAlert." This is an alert system for those patients who actually use this on-line pharmacy as their drugstore. It provides up-to-date information about new adverse drug reactions, interactions, or withdrawals of your particular medications. You may want to ask your personal pharmacy if they provide a similar service. Now that you know the dynamic

changes occurring with medication use today, being informed and having an alert system are definitely important aspects of drug safety.

www.PDR.net is also a great site for easy access to drug information. Simply type in the drug name in which you are interested, then click on the name of the drug to get valuable information.

Notes

CHAPTER 1
1. J. Lazarou, B. Pomeranz, and P. Corey, "Incidence of adverse drug reactions in hospitalized patients," *JAMA,* 279 (1998), 1200–05.
2. Department of Health and Human Services, *Health United States 1996–97 and Injury Chartbook* (July 1997) and *The 10 Leading Causes of Death* (DHHS Publication No. PHS 97–1232), 964.
3. D. Bates, J. Cullen, N. Laird, et al., "Incidence of adverse drug events and potential adverse drug events," *JAMA,* 274 (1995), 29–34.
4. Ibid.
5. Ibid.
6. K. M. Nelson and R. L. Talbert, "Drug-Related Hospital Admissions," *Pharmacy Practice Insights* (1994) 701–7.
7. T. Einarson, "Drug-related hospital admissions," *Annals of Pharmacotherapy*, 27 (1993), 832–40.
8. D. Bates, L. Leape, and S. Petrycki, "Incidence and preventability of adverse drug events in hospitalized adults," *Journal of General Internal Medicine,* 8 (June 1993), 289–94.
9. D. Phillips, N. Christenfeld, and L. Glynn, "Increase in U.S. medication-error deaths between 1983 and 1993," *Lancet,* 351 (1998), 643–44.
10. Ibid.

CHAPTER 2
1. U.S. Food and Drug Administration, *Consumer Special Report: Benefit vs. Risk: How CDER Approves Drugs* (January 1995).
2. Ibid.
3. V. Orlando, "The FDA's accelerated approval process: does the pharmaceutical industry have adequate incentives for self-regulation?" *American Journal of Law & Medicine & Ethics,* 25 (1999), 543–68.
4. Ibid.
5. G. J. Annas and S. Elias, "Thalidomide and the *Titanic:* reconstructing the technology tragedies of the twentieth century," *American Journal of Public Health,* 89 (1999), 98–101.
6. Ibid.
7. Ibid.
8. The FDA has since approved thalidomide for prescription use in patients who suffer from *erythema nodosum leprosum*, a severe skin condition found in patients with Hansen's disease (leprosy). The FDA has announced that thalidomide will be among the most tightly restricted drugs in the history of the United States—but a nagging fear remains, due to the fact that physicians can now use thalidomide "off-label." In other words, physicians may choose to use this drug for reasons other than strictly for patients who have leprosy. For example, thalidomide is also very effective in healing mouth ulcers in patients with AIDS. For further discussion on off-label drugs, see Chapter 6.
9. U.S. Food and Drug Administration, *Benefit vs. Risk* (1995).
10. Orlando, "The FDA's accelerated approval process."

236

11. Ibid.
12. K. Flieger, U.S. Food & Drug Administration, *Consumer Special Report: Testing Drugs in People* (July-August 1994 FDA Consumer), www.fda.gov/fdac/special/newdrug/testing.html.
13. Ibid.
14. Ibid.
15. U.S. Food and Drug Administration: *Prescription Drug User Fee Act, PDUFA Background Information* (January 21, 2001), http://www.fda.gov/oc/pdufa2/meeting2000/background.html.

CHAPTER 3
1. U.S. Food and Drug Administration: *Prescription Drug User Fee Act, PDUFA Background Information* (2000), http://www.fda.gov/oc/pdufa2/meeting 2000/background.html.
2. *Vital Signs.* "The Bottom Line on Drug Spending," GlaxoWellcome Public Policy and Advocacy Department, Vol. 5, No. 2.
3. U.S. Food and Drug Administration: *Prescription Drug User Fee Act*
4. L. Thompson, "User Fees for Faster Drug Reviews: Are They Helping or Hurting the Public Health?" *FDA Consumer Magazine,* (September-October 2000), http://www.fda.gov/fdacfeatures/2000/500_pdufa.html.
5. G. Binder, "Pharmaceutical provisions of the FDA Modernization Act of 1997: one year and counting," *Current Opinion in Biotechnology,* 10 (1999), 303–6.
6. Ibid.
7. Thompson, "User Fees for Faster Drug Reviews."
8. Ibid.
9. Ibid.
10. Ibid.
11. U.S. Food and Drug Administration: *Prescription Drug User Fee Act.*
12. R. Merrill, "Modernizing the FDA: an incremental revolution," *Health Affairs,* 18 (1999), 96–111.
13. Ibid.
14. M. Friedman, "Changes at FDA may speed drug-approval process and increase off-label use," *Journal of the National Cancer Institute,* 90 (1998), 805–7.
15. Ibid.
16. D. Willman, "How a New Policy Led to Seven Deadly Drugs," *Los Angeles Times,* 20 December 2000, http://www.latimes.com/cgi-bin/print.cgi
17. M. Reh, "FDA to require pediatric studies for drugs commonly used in children," *American Journal Health-Systems Pharmacists,* 56 (1999), 203.
18. Friedman, "Changes at FDA."
19. Merrill, "Modernizing the FDA."
20. K. Flieger, U.S. Food and Drug Administration, *Consumer Special Report: FDA Finds New Ways to Speed Treatments to Patients* (October 1993), 15–18.
21. U.S. Food and Drug Administration, *FDA and Stakeholders Public Meeting: Executive Summary,* (October 19, 2000), http://www.fda.gov/oc/pdufa2/meeting2000/meeting 2000summ.html.

CHAPTER 4
1. D. Willman, "Drug after Drug, Warnings Ignored," *Los Angeles Times,* 20 December 2000, http://www.latimes.com/health/consumer/connews/20001220/t000121361.html.
2. Center for Health Policy Research, George Washington University, "Time to Act on Drug Safety," *JAMA,* 279 (1998), 1571–73.

3. M. Friedman, J. Woodcock, M. Lumpkin, et al., "The safety of newly approved medicines: do recent market removals mean there is a problem?" *JAMA*, 281 (1999), 1728–34.

4. P. Montague, "Prescription Drugs That Kill: Another Kind of Drug Problem," *Consumer Law Page* (2000), http://consumerlawpage.com/article/drugs_that_kill.shtml.

5. I. Oransky, "Doctors Step Out; Drug Salesmen Step In," *USA Today*, 5 July 2001, 11A.

6. National Academy of Sciences, *Report of the International Conference on Adverse Reactions Reporting Systems*, Washington, D.C. (1971).

7. Center for Health Policy Research, George Washington University, "Time to Act on Drug Safety."

8. Ibid.

9. Ibid.

10. Montague, "Prescription Drugs That Kill."

11. D. Willman, "How a New Policy Led to Seven Deadly Drugs," *Los Angeles Times*, 20 December 2000, http://www.latimes.com/cgi-bin/print.cgi.

12. Center for Health Policy Research, "Time to Act on Drug Safety."

13. Willman, "How a New Policy Led to Seven Deadly Drugs."

14. K. E. Lasser, et al., "Timing of New Black Box Warnings and Withdrawals for Prescription Medications," *JAMA*, 287, no. 17 (May 1, 2002).

CHAPTER 5

1. D. Willman, "The Rise and Fall of the Killer Drug Rezulin," *Los Angeles Times*, 4 June 2000, http://www.latimes.com/news/nation/reports/rezulin/lat_rezulin000604.htm.

2. D. Willman, "Drug Maker Hired NIH Researcher," *Los Angeles Times*, 7 December 1998, http://www.latimes.com/news/nation/reports/rezulin/lat_main981207.htm.

3. Ibid.

4. Ibid.

5. Willman, "The Rise and Fall of the Killer Drug Rezulin."

6. Ibid.

7. Ibid.

8. A. Cifaldi, "Litigating Rezulin Cases," Diss. *ATLA's Litigating Rezulin Cases* (Chicago, IL, 2000).

9. D. Willman, "Rezulin's Effect on Heart Was Also Seen as Concern," *Los Angeles Times*, 26 March 2000, http://www.latimes.com/news/nation/reports/rezulin/lat_heart000326.htm.

10. Cifaldi, "Litigating Rezulin Cases."

11. Willman, "Rezulin's Effect on Heart."

12. C. Zevitas, "Diabetes Drug Could Spur Next Big Pharmaceutical Litigation," http://www.lweekly.com/diabetes.cfm.

13. SE Inzucchi, DG Maggs, et al., "Efficacy and metabolic effects of metformin and troglitazone in type II diabetes mellitus," NEJM, 338 (March 26, 1998): 13.

14. S. Schwartz, P. Raskin, et al., "Effect of troglitazone in insulin-treated patients with type II diabetes mellitus", NEJM, 338 (March 26, 1998): 13.

15. H. Imura, "A novel antidiabetic drug, Troglitazone—reason for hope and concern," NEJM, 338, no. 13 (March 26, 1998).

16. Willman, "Drug Maker Hired NIH Researcher."

17. D. Willman, "Second of Two Parts: Drug Maker Hired NIH Researcher," *Los Angeles Times*, 7 December 1998, http://www.latimes.com/news/nation/reports/rezulin/lat_main981207.

18. Allen Spiegel, director of the National Institute of Diabetes, recently released the

results of the Diabetes Prevention Program. This study involved more than three thousand overweight patients who had a prediabetic condition called *impaired glucose intolerance*. This means that their blood sugars were elevated above the normal range but were still not high enough to be labeled diabetic. They followed these patients for three years (and actually cut the study short by one year because of the impressive results). There were three different groups: the control group, which received a placebo; a group that received a drug called metformin—Glucophage—twice daily along with information on diet and exercise; and a group that received no medication but was instructed in changes of diet and moderate (thirty minutes daily) exercise. Results: The metformin group members decreased their risk of developing full-blown diabetes by 31 percent. The diet and exercise group members decreased their risk of developing diabetes by 58 percent (they were on no medication and they lost an average of ten to fifteen pounds).

19. Willman.
20. Cifaldi, "Litigating Rezulin Cases."
21. Watkins, Whitcomb "Hepatic dysfunction associated with Troglitazone," NEJM, Letter to the Editor (March 26, 1998), 916–17.
22. Cifaldi.
23. Willman, "The Rise and Fall of the Killer Drug Rezulin."
24. Cifaldi, "Litigating Rezulin Cases."
25. Ibid.
26. Willman, "The Rise and Fall of the Killer Drug Rezulin."
27. Ibid.
28. Ibid.
29. Ibid. (Note: The inner workings of the FDA were only made known on this story because David Willman conducted an aggressive investigational report for the *Los Angeles Times*. I believe Willman's tenacity in reporting the different aspects of this story to the public deserves the most credit for getting Rezulin off the market.)
30. Willman.
31. Ibid.
32. Ibid.
33. Willman, "Drug Maker Hired NIH Researcher."
34. Willman, "FDA Official Says Lessons Have Been Learned from Rezulin," *Los Angeles Times*, 4 June 2000.

Chapter 6
1. Center for Health Policy Research, "Time to Act on Drug Safety," *JAMA*, 279 (1998).
2. "Propulsid Used to Treat Babies' Heartburn," *Propulsid Legal Help* (2000), www.propulsid-legalhelp.com.
3. D. Willman, "Drug after Drug, Warnings Ignored." *Los Angeles Times*, 20 December 2000.
4. Ibid.
5. W. Smalley, D. Shatin, et al., "Contraindicated use of cisapride," *JAMA*, 284, no. 23 (December 20, 2000).
6. Willman, "How a New Policy Led to Seven Deadly Drugs," *Los Angeles Times*, 20 December 2000, http://www.latimes.com/cgi-bin/print.cgi.
7. Willman, "Drug after Drug, Warnings Ignored."
8. Willman, "How a New Policy Led to Seven Deadly Drugs."
9. Willman, "Drug after Drug, Warnings Ignored."
10. Ibid.
11. Willman, "How a New Policy Led to Seven Deadly Drugs."

12. Smalley, et al., "Contraindicated Use of Cisapride."
13. Ibid.
14. Ibid.
15. Ibid.
16. Willman, "Drug after Drug, Warnings Ignored."
17. "Prescription Pain-reliever Duract Recalled Following Four Deaths," *The Shawnee News-Star Online*, 23 June 1998, http://www.news-star.com/stories/062398/lif_prescription.html.
18. J. L. Miller, "Drug review and postmarketing surveillance programs are sound, but systems approach to risk management is needed, says FDA," *American Journal of Heath Syst Pharm* 1999 Jul 1; 56 (13):1294, 6.
19. T. Moore, "Time to Act on Drug Safety." *JAMA*, 279, no. 19 (May 20, 1998).
20. S. Sternberg, "Lawsuits: Drug Development's Side Effect." *USA Today*, 12 January 2000.
21. D. Kessler, "Introducing MedWatch: a new approach to reporting medication and device adverse effects and product problems," *JAMA*, 269 (1993), 2765–68.
22. Ibid.

CHAPTER 7
1. "Bayer Pulls Anti-Cholesterol Drug," *Associated Press Online*, 23 August 2001, http://www.baycol-com/press_articles.htm.
2. Ibid.
3. Ibid.
4. Ibid.
5. Ibid.
6. "The Baycol Recall: How Safe Is Your Statin?" *Washington Post*, 14 August 2001, http://www.baycol-com/press_articles.htm.
7. "Bayer Pulls Anti-Cholesterol Drug."
8. "The Baycol Recall: How Safe Is Your Statin?"
9. P. Hilts, "Drug's Problems Raise Questions on Warnings," *New York Times*, 21 August 2001.
10. Ibid.
11. *Physicians' Desk Reference*, warnings and recommendations found under the statin drugs—Lipitor, Zocor, etc.

CHAPTER 8
1. Centers for Disease Control and Prevention, "Cardiac Valvulopathy Associated with Exposure to Fenfluramine or Dexfenfluramine: U.S. Department of Health and Human Services Interim Public Health Recommendations," *Morbidity and Mortality Weekly Report*, 46 (November 1997), 1061–66.
2. Ibid.
3. Ibid.
4. Ibid.
5. Ibid.
6. Ibid.
7. Ibid.
8. Ibid.
9. American Society of Health-System Pharmacists, "Snapshot of Medication Use in the U. S.," December 2000.
10. D. Willman, "Drug after Drug, Warnings Ignored."

11. Ibid.
12. Ibid.
13. Ibid.
14. Ibid.
15. Ibid.
16. A. Rankin, "Non-sedating antihistamines and cardiac arrhythmia," *Lancet*, 350 (1997), 1115–16.
17. Ibid.

CHAPTER 9

1. P. A. Frisk, J. Cooper, and N. Campbell, "Community-hospital pharmacist detection of drug-related problems upon patient admission to small hospitals," *American Journal of Hospital Pharmacists*, 34 (1977), 738–42.
2. Bates, et al., "Incidence and preventability of adverse drug events in hospitalized adults," *Journal of General Internal Medicine*, 8 (June 1993), 289–94.
3. Ibid.
4. Ibid.
5. Ibid.
6. D. Phillips, et al., "Increase in U.S. medication-error deaths between 1983 and 1993," *Lancet* 351 (1998), 643–44.
7. Ibid.
8. Todd Weber, "2000 Annual Session Press Briefing: Antibiotic Resistance" (April 14, 2000).
9. Ibid.
10. Ibid.
11. L. Hickling, "The Rise of Antibiotic-Resistant Bacteria" (November 3, 2000), www.drkoop.com Health News.
12. L. McCaig, R. Blesser, and J. Hughes, "Trends in antimicrobial prescribing rates for children and adolescents," *JAMA*, 287 (2002), 3096–3102.
13. Ibid.
14. J. Perz, A. Craig, and C. Coffey, "Changes in antibiotic prescribing for children after a community-wide campaign," *JAMA*, 287 (2002), 3103–09.
15. Ibid.
16. S. Bedell, S. Jabbour, and R. Goldberg, "Discrepancies in the use of medications," *Arch Intern Medicine*, 160 (2000), 2129–34.

CHAPTER 10

1. K. Nelson, R. Talbert, FCCP, "Drug-related hospital admissions," *Pharmacy Practice Insights* (1994), 701–07.
2. Writing Group for the Women's Health Initiative Investigators, "Risks and Benefits of Estrogen Plus Progestin in Healthy Postmenopausal Women," *JAMA*, 299, no. 3 (July 17, 2002).
3. Kaufman, D., Kelly, J., Rosenberg, L., et al., "Recent Patterns of Medication Use in the Ambulatory Adult Population of the United States: The Slone Survey." *JAMA*, 287 (2002), 337-44.
4. Smith, S., "Dangerous Drug Mishaps," *Ladies Home Journal*—Online, May, 1999.
5. Ibid.
6. Ibid.
7. "Warning About Mixing Prescription Drugs Not Always Given," *Atlanta Journal Constitution*, 19 August 1996, http://www.pendulum.org/articles/mising_meds.htm.

CHAPTER 11

1. Partnership for Self-Care; http://www.pharmacyandyou.org/selfcare/factsheet.html.
2. T. Klepser and M. Klepser, "Unsafe and Potentially Safe Herbal Therapies," *American Journal of American Health-System Pharmacists,* 56 (1999), 125-38.
3. J. Kirchner, "Improper Dosing of Over the Counter Medications Given by Caregivers," *American Family Physician* (February 1, 1998), http://www.findarticles.com/cf_dsl/m3225/n3_v57/20298020/pl/article.jhtml.
4. Ashcraft & Gerel, LLP, "Claims for Stroke Resulting from Phenylpropanolamine or PPA in Over-the-Counter Diet Drugs and Cold Medications," http://www.ashcraftandgerel.com/ppa.html.
5. Ibid.
6. Center for Drug Evaluation and Research, "Food And Drug Administration, Science Background, Safety of Phenylpropanolamine," (6 November2000), http://www.fda.gov/cder/drug/infopage/ppa/science.htm.
7. Ibid.
8. Ibid.
9. Ibid.
10. M. M. Wolfe and D. R. Lichtenstein, et al., "Gastrointestinal Toxicity of Nonsteroidal Antiinflammatory Drugs," *New England Journal of Medicine,* 340, no. 24 (June 17, 1999), 1888–89.
11. Ibid.
12. M. N. Dukes, ed., *Meyler's Side Effects of Drugs,* 14th ed. (Elsevier 2000), 252.
13. Ibid.

CHAPTER 12

1. T. Klepser and M. Klepser, "Unsafe and potentially safe herbal therapies," *American Journal of American Health-System Pharmacists,* 56 (1999), 125–38.
2. Ibid.
3. Ibid.
4. Ibid.
5. Ibid.
6. M. Ang-Lee, J. Moss, and C. Yaun, "Herbal medicines and perioperative care," *JAMA,* 286 (2001), 208–16.
7. Haller, Benowitz, "Adverse cardiovascular and central nervous system events associated with the dietary supplements containing Ephedra alkaloids," *NEJM,* December 21, 2000.
8. Klepser, "Unsafe and potentially safe herbal therapies."
9. Ibid.
10. Ibid.
11. Ibid.
12. Ibid.
13. Ibid.
14. Ibid.
15. A. D. Kaye, R.C. Clarke, et al., "Herbal Medications: current trends in anesthesiology," *Journal of Clinical Anesthesia,* 12 (2000): 468–710.
16. Ang-Lee, et al., "Herbal medicines and perioperative Care."
17. E. Hawkins, "And the Good Herb Taketh Away," *Nutrition Science News,* 4 (1999), 482–83.
18. Ang-Lee.
19. Ibid.

20. R. Roundtree, "Herbs and Drugs for Your Heart: Sorting Out What's Safe," *Herbs for Health* (November/December 1999), 28–29.
21. Hawkins, "And the Good Herb Taketh Away."

CHAPTER 13
1. A. Rankin, "Non-Sedating Antihistamines and Cardiac Arrhythmia," *The Lancet*, 350 (1997), 1115-16.
2. "Drug Studies to Face Scrutiny by Journals," *USA Today*, 6 August 2001, 4D.

CHAPTER 14
1. M. Nelson, et al., "A systematic review of predictors of maintenance of nomotension after withdrawal of antihypertensive drugs," *American Journal of Hypertension*, 14 (2001), 98–105.
2. The Diabetes Prevention Program Research Group, "The Diabetes Prevention Program," Diabetes Care, 22, no. 4 (April, 1999).
3. D. Ludwig, "The glycemic index: physiological mechanisms relating to obesity, diabetes, and cardiovascular disease," *JAMA*, 287 (2002), 2414–23.
4. Ibid.
5. Ibid.
6. Ibid.
7. C. D. Gardner and H. C. Draemer, "Monounsaturated versus polyunsaturated dietary fat and serum lipids. A meta-analysis," *Arterioscler Thromb Vasc Biol*, 15 (1995) 1917.
8. Issued by the surgeon general of the United States as a result of having a modest exercise program.
9. C. Davies, "Oxidative stress: the paradox of aerobic life," *Biochem Soc Symp*, 61 (1995), 1-31.

Bibliography

Agency for Healthcare Research and Quality. "Medical Errors: The Scope of the Problem." Fact sheet, Publication No. AHRQ 00-P037, 2001.<http://www.ahcpr.gov/qual/errback.htm>.

Ajayi, F., H. Sun, and J. Perry. "Adverse Drug Reactions: A Review of Relevant Factors." *Journal of Clinical Pharmacology* 40 (2000): 1093–1101.

American Society of Health-System Pharmacists. "Snapshot of Medication Use in the U.S.," December 2000.

Anello, C. "Emerging and Recurrent Issues in Drug Development." *Statistics in Medicine* 18 (1999): 2301–9.

Ang-Lee, M., J. Moss, and C. Yaun. "Herbal Medicines and Perioperative Care." *JAMA* 286 (2001): 208–16.

Annas, G. J., and S. Elias. "Thalidomide and the Titanic: Reconstructing the Technology Tragedies of the Twentieth Century." *American Journal of Public Health* 89 (1999): 98–101.

Ashcraft & Gerel, LLP. "Claims for Stroke Resulting from Phenylpropanolamine or PPA in Over-the-Counter Diet Drugs and Cold Medications."<http://www.ashcraftandgerel.com/ppa.html>.

Ashish, K., et al. "Identifying Adverse Drug Events." *Journal of the American Medical Informatics Association* 5 (1998): 305–14.

Bates, D., et al. "The Costs of Adverse Drug Events in Hospitalized Patients." *JAMA* 277 (1997): 307–11.

Bates, D., et al. "Incidence of Adverse Drug Events and Potential Adverse Drug Events." *JAMA* 274 (1995): 29–34.

Bates, D., L. Leape, and S. Petrycki. "Incidence and Preventability of Adverse Drug Events in Hospitalized Adults." *Journal of General Internal Medicine* 8 (June 1993): 289–94.

Baumann, J. "Doctors Warned to Be Wary of New Drugs." *British Medical Journal* 324 (2002): 1113.

"The Baycol Recall: How Safe Is Your Statin?" *Washington Post,* 14 August 2001. <http://www.baycol-com/press_articles.htm>.

"Bayer Pulls Anti-Cholesterol Drug," Associated Press Online, 23 August 2001. <http://www.baycol-com/press_articles.htm>.

Bedell, S., S. Jabbour, and R. Goldberg. "Discrepancies in the Use of Medications." *Arch Intern Medicine* 160 (2000): 2129–34.

Binder, G. "Pharmaceutical Provisions of the FDA Modernization Act of 1997: One Year and Counting." *Current Opinion in Biotechnology* 10 (1999): 303–6.

Brewer, T., and G. Colditz. "Postmarketing Surveillance and Adverse Drug Reactions: Current Perspectives and Future Needs." *JAMA* 281 (1999): 824–29.

Caranasos, G., R. Stewart, and L. Cluff. "Drug-Induced Illness Leading to Hospitalization." *JAMA* 228 (1974): 713–17.

Carbonin, P., et al. "Is Age an Independent Risk Factor of Adverse Drug Reactions in

Hospitalized Medical Patients?" *Journal of the American Geriatrics Society* 39 (1991): 1093–99.

Cassell, G. "Senator Frist and Senator Kennedy Congressional Round Table Discussion on Antimicrobial Resistance." *American Society for Microbiology,* Diss. (2001). <http://www.asmusa.org/pasrc/antibioticres.htm>.

Center for Drug Evaluation and Research. "Food and Drug Administration, Science Background, Safety of Phenylpropanolamine," 6 November 2000. <http://www.fda.gov/cder/drug/infopage/ppa/science.htm>.

Center for Health Policy Research, George Washington University. "Time to Act on Drug Safety." *JAMA* 279 (1998): 1571–73.

Centers for Disease Control and Prevention. "Cardiac Valvulopathy Associated with Exposure to Fenfluramine or Dexfenfluramine: U.S. Department of Health and Human Services Interim Public Health Recommendations." *Morbidity and Mortality Weekly Report* 46 (14 November 1997): 1061–66.

Chyka, P. "How Many Deaths Occur Annually from Adverse Drug Reactions in the United States." *American Journal of Medicine* 109 (2000): 122–30.

Cifaldi, A. "Litigating Rezulin Cases." Report first given at *ATLA's Litigating Rezulin Cases,* Chicago, IL, 2000.

Classen, D., et al. "Adverse Drug Events in Hospitalized Patients." *JAMA* 227 (1997): 301–6.

Classen, D., et al. "Computerized Surveillance of Adverse Drug Events in Hospital Patients." *JAMA* 266 (1991): 2847–51.

Cobert, B., and J. Silvey. "The Internet and Drug Safety: What Are the Implications for Pharmacovigilance?" *Drug Safety* 20 (1999): 95–107.

Cullen, D., et al. "The Incident Reporting System Does Not Detect Adverse Drug Events." *Journal on Quality Improvement* 21 (1995): 541–48.

Department of Clinical and Quality Analysis Partners Healthcare Systems, Boston, Mass. "Drugs and Adverse Drug Reactions: How Worried Should We Be?" *JAMA* 279 (1998): 1216–17.

Department of Food and Nutrition at ViaHealth. "Taking Prescription Drugs and Herbal Supplements: Known Interactions to Avoid," 2001. <http://www.viahealth.org/nutrition/interactions.htm>.

Department of Health and Human Services: Food and Drug Administration. "Dissemination of Information on Unapproved/New Uses for Marketed Drugs, Biologics, and Devices." *Federal Register* 63 (1998): 64556–87.

Department of Health and Human Services. *Health United States 1996–97 and Injury Chartbook* (July 1997) and *The 10 Leading Causes of Death* (DHHS Publication No. PHS 97–1232), 964.

Department of Health and Human Services. "List of Drug Products That Have Been Withdrawn or Removed from the Market for Reasons of Safety or Effectiveness. Food and Drug Administration, HHS. Final Rule." *Federal Register* 64 (1999): 10944–47.

"Drug and Herbal Interactions." *Spring net—CE Connection.* (2001). <http://www.springnet.com/ce/cam_mod2.htm>.

———. "Drug Maker Hired NIH Researcher." *Los Angeles Times,* 7 December 1998. <http://www.latimes.com/news/nation/reports/rezulin/lat_main981207.htm>.

"Drug Review and Postmarketing Surveillance Programs Are Sound, but Systems Approach to Risk Management Is Needed, Says FDA." *American Journal of Health Systems Pharmacists* 56 (1999): 1294, 1946.

"Drug Studies to Face Scrutiny by Journals." *USA TODAY*, A Better Life: Health, Education & Science, 6 August 2001.

Einarson, T. "Drug-Related Hospital Admissions." *Annals of Pharmacotherapy* 27 (1993): 832–40.

"Failure to Recognize Adverse Drug Reactions Despite Warnings." *Adverse Drug Reaction Toxicology Review* 18 (1998): 1–3.

"FDA Drug-Review, Surveillance Processes Under Scrutiny." *American Journal Health-System Pharmacists* 56 (1999): 405–8.

"FDA Treads Delicate Line Between Safety and Speed." *Oncology,* 13, 16.

Flieger, K. U.S. Food & Drug Administration. *Consumer Special Report: FDA Finds New Ways to Speed Treatments to Patients,* October 1993, 15–18.

———. *FDA and Stakeholders Public Meeting: Executive Summary,* 19 October 2000. <http://www.fda.gov/oc/pdufa2/meeting2000/meeting2000summ.html>.

———. "FDA Announces Withdrawal of Fenfluramine and Dexfenfluramine (Fen-Phen)," 15 September 1997.<http://www.fda.gov/cder/news/phen/fenphenpr81597.htm>.

———. "FDA Approval and Delay in Withdrawing Rezulin Probed." *Los Angeles Times,* 16 August 2000. <http://www.latimes.com/news/nation/reports/rezulinlat_fda00816.htm>.

———. "FDA Official Says Lessons Have Been Learned from Rezulin." *Los Angeles Times,* 4 June 2000.<http://www.latimes.com/news/nation/reports/rezulin/lat_rezside000604.htm>.

———. "FDA Post-Mortem Finds Drug Approval Problems." *Los Angeles Times,* 16 November 2000. <http://www.latimes.com/news/nation/reports/rezulinlat_fda001116.htm>.

———. *FDA Talk Paper: Bayer Voluntarily Withdraws Baycol,* 8 August 2001, T01–34.

———. *FDA Talk Paper: Wyeth-Ayerst Laboratories Announces the Withdrawal of Duract from the Market,* June 1998. <http://www.fda.gov/bbs/topics/ANSWERS/ANS00879.html>.

Flieger, K. U.S. Food & Drug Administration. *Consumer Special Report: Testing Drugs in People,* 1995, www.fda.gov/fdac/special/newdrug/testing.html.

Fowler, M. "An Overview of Diabetes, Rezulin, and the Liver." *ATLA's Litigating Rezulin Cases,* Chicago, IL, June 2000.

Friedman, M. "Changes at FDA May Speed Drug-approval process and Increase Off-Label Use." *Journal of the National Cancer Institute* 90 (1998): 805–7.

Friedman, M., et al. "The Safety of Newly Approved Medicines: Do Recent Market Removals Mean There Is a Problem?" *JAMA* 281 (1999): 1728–34.

Friend, T. "Defusing Dangerous Drug Interactions." *USA Today,* 1997. <http://www.usatoday.com/hotlines/pharm97/hotphr01.htm>.

Frisk, P. A., J. Cooper, and N. Campbell. "Community-Hospital Pharmacist Detection of Drug-Related Problems upon Patient Admission to Small Hospitals," *American Journal of Hospital Pharmacist* 34 (1977): 738–42.

Gardner, C. D., and H. C. Draemer. "Monounsaturated Versus Polyunsaturated Dietary Fat and Serum Lipids: A Meta-Analysis." *Arteriosclerosis, Thrombosis, and Vascular Biology* 15 (1995): 1917–27.

Generali, J. "Avoiding Drug Interactions." *American Family Physician,* March 2000. <http://www.findarticles.com/m3225/6_61/61432857/pl/article.jhtml>.

Glaxo Wellcome: Public Policy & Advocacy Department. "Vital Signs: The Bottom Line on Drug Spending," 1998. (A letter to the author).

Goldberg, R. "Breaking Up the FDA's Medical Information Monopoly." <http://www.cato.org/pubs/reglation/reg18n2c.html>.

Golodner, L. "The U.S. Food and Drug Administration Modernization Act of 1997: Impact on Consumers." *Clinical Therapeutics* 20 (1998): C20–C25.

Graham, D., et al. "Liver Enzyme Monitoring in Patients Treated with Troglitazone." *JAMA*

286 (2001): 831–33.

Haller, C. A., and N. L. Benowitz. "Adverse Cardiovascular and Central Nervous System Events Associated with the Dietary Supplements Containing Ephedra Alkaloids." *New England Journal of Medicine,* 21 December 2000.

Hanan, T. "Detecting Adverse Drug Reactions to Improve Patient Outcomes." *International Journal of Medical Information* 55 (1999): 61–64.

Hawkins, E. "And the Good Herb Taketh Away." *Nutrition Science News* 4 (1999): 482–83.<http://www.medscape.com/Medscape/features/newsbeat/2000/1100/PPA.html>.

Hayward, R., and T. Hofer. "Estimating Hospital Deaths Due to Medical Errors." *JAMA* 286 (2001): 415–20.

Henkel, J., U.S. Food and Drug Administration. *Part 2: User Fees to Fund Faster Reviews,* October 1993. <http://www.fda.gov/bbs/topics/CONSUMER/CON0257d.html>.

"Herbal Poisoning: Cautions About Herbs." *KSL TV,* 2001. <http://www.ksl.com/TV/series/herb/page1.htm>.

———. "Herbal Supplements May Be Dangerous." *Association of Trial Lawyers of America,* Reprinted from TRIAL 42, November 1999.

Hershel, J. "The Discovery of Drug-Induced Illness." *New England Journal of Medicine* 296 (1977): 481–85.

Herxheimer, A. "Possible Harm from Drugs: When and How to Inform Doctors and Users." <http://www.aston.ac.uk/pharmacy/cebp/cpharm/P'vig%20Anka%20R3.htm>.

Hickling, L. "The Rise of Antibiotic-Resistant Bacteria." *drkoop.com Health News,* 3 November 2000. <http://mc.drkoop.com/news/stories/2000/nov/03_bacteria.html?nl=mc&scr=top&dt=110900>.

Hilts, P. "Drug's Problems Raise Questions on Warnings." *New York Times,* 21 August 2001. <http://www.nytimes.com/2001/08/21/health/policy/21DRUG.html?ei=5007&en=do8dff82>.

———. "How a New Policy Led to Seven Deadly Drugs." *Los Angeles Times,* 20 December 2000. <http://www.latimes.com/cgi-bin/print.cgi>.

Imura, H. "A Novel Antidiabetic Drug, Troglitazone—Reason for Hope and Concern." *New England Journal of Medicine* 338 (March 1998): 908–9.

"Increased Antibiotic Use Can Lead to Drug Resistance." *Doctor's Guide to the Internet,* 1997. <http://www.pslgroup.com/dg/38FEA.htm>.

International Communications Research for the American Society of Health-System Pharmacists. "Snapshot of Medication Use in the U.S.," December 2000, 1–9.

Jameson, J., and G. VanNoord. "Pharmacotherapy Consultation on Polypharmacy Patients in Ambulatory Care." *Annual of Pharmacotherapy* 35 (2001): 835–40.

Joseph, J. "Double-Edged Sword of Drugs." *ABC News,* 13 April 1998. <http://abcnews.go.com/sections/living/DailyNews/drugreactions980413.html>.

Karch, F., et al. "Commentary—Adverse Drug Reactions—a Matter of Opinion." *Clinical Pharmacology and Therapeutics* 19 (1976): 489–92.

Kaufman, D., et al. "Recent Patterns of Medication Use in the Ambulatory Adult Population of the United States: The Slone Survey," *JAMA* 287 (2002): 337–44.

Kaye, A. D., et al. "Herbal Medications: Current Trends in Anesthesiology." *Journal of Clinical Anesthesia* 12 (2000): 468–71.

Kessler, D. "Introducing MedWatch: A New Approach to Reporting Medication and Device Adverse Effects and Product Problems." *JAMA* 269 (1993): 2765–68.

Kirchner, J. "Improper Dosing of Over the Counter Medications Given by Caregivers," *American Family Physician,* 1 February 1998. <http://www.findarticles.com/cf_dsl/m3225/n3_v57/20298020/pl/article.jhtml>.

BIBLIOGRAPHY

Kleinke, J. "Is the FDA Approving Drugs Too Fast?" *British Medical Journal* 317 (1998): 899.

Klepser, T., and M. Klepser. "Unsafe and Potentially Safe Herbal Therapies." *American Journal of American Health-System Pharmacists* 56 (1999): 125–38.

Knapp, D., J. Rovinson, and A. Fritt. *Annual Adverse Drug Experience Report: 1995.* Food and Drug Administration. 1–18.

Knight, S., et al. "Iatrogenic Illness on a General Medical Service at a University Hospital." *New England Journal of Medicine* 304 (1981): 638–42.

Kolata, G., and E. Andrews. "Baycol: In the News: Anticholesterol Drug Pulled After Link to 31 Deaths." *Early, Ludwick, Sweeney, and Strauss Law,* 2001. <http://www.elslaw-baycol_news_8-0-01.htm>.

LaCalamita, S. "Top 10 Reasons for Not Reporting Adverse Drug Reactions." *Hospital Pharmacy* 30 (1995): 245–46.

Lakshmanan, M., Hershey, C., and Breslau, D. "Hospital Admissions Caused by Iatrogenic Disease." Department of Medicine, Western Reserve University (1986). Reprints of this article can be obtained by writing the National Institutes of Health—Clinical Endocrinology Branch, Bethesda, Md.

Lasser, K. E., et al. "Timing of New Black Box Warnings and Withdrawals for Prescription Medications." *JAMA* 287 (May 2002).

"Lawsuit Filed Against Bayer." *Los Angeles Times,* 14 August 2001. <http://www.latimes.com/features/health/ wire/sns-ap-bayer-lawsuit0814aug14.story>.

Lazarou, J., B. Pomeranz, and P. Corey. "Incidence of Adverse Drug Reactions in Hospitalized Patients." *JAMA* 279 (1998): 1200–05.

"Legal-Medical Resources for People Who Took Rezulin." *Rezulin Newsletter,* 13 April 2001. <http://www.rezulinnewsletter.com/history_of_rezulin_fda_and_recall.htm>.

———. "List of Drug Products That Have Been Withdrawn or Removed from the Market for Reasons of Safety or Effectiveness." *Federal Register* 63 (1998): 54082–89.

Ludwig, D. "The Glycemic Index: Physiological Mechanisms Relating to Obesity, Diabetes, and Cardiovascular Disease." *JAMA* 287 (2002): 2414–23.

Lumpkin, M., Center for Drug Evaluation and Research. "Reports of Valvular Heart Disease in Patients Receiving Concomitant Fenfluramine and Phentermine." Letter. *FDA Public Health Advisory,* August 1997. <http://www.fda.gov/cder/news/phen/phenfen.htm>.

Lurie, P., and L. Sasich. "Safety of FDA-Approved Drugs." *JAMA* 282 (1999): 2297–98.

Lurie, P., and S. Wolfe. "FDA Medical Officers Report Lower Standards Permit Dangerous Drug Approvals." *Public Citizen: FDA Medical Officers Survey,* 1999. <http://www.citizen.org/hrg/publications/FDAsurvey/FDAsurvey.htm>.

McCaig, L., R. Blesser, and J. Hughes, "Trends in Antimicrobial Prescribing Rates for Children and Adolescents." *JAMA* 287 (2002): 3096–102.

McNeil, J., E. Grabsch, and M. McDonald. "Postmarketing Surveillance: Strengths and Limitations. The Flucloxacillin-Dicloxacillin Story." *Medical Journal Australia* 170 (1999): 270–73.

Merrill, R. "Modernizing the FDA: An Incremental Revolution." *Health Affairs* 18 (1999): 96–111.

Miller, J. L. "Drug Review and Postmarketing Surveillance Programs Are Sound, but Systems Approach to Risk Management Is Needed, Says FDA." *American Journal of Health System Pharmacists,* 1 July 1999, 56(13):1294, 6.

Mitchell, A., et al. "Drug Utilization and Reported Adverse Reactions in Hospitalized Children." *American Journal of Epidemiology* 110 (1979): 196–204.

Mitchell, P., J. Sheehan, and S. Shapiro. "Adverse Drug Reactions in Children Leading to

Hospital Admission." *American Academy of Pediatrics* 82 (1998): 24–29.

Miwa, J., et al. "Value of Epidemiologic Studies in Determining the True Incidence of Adverse Events." *Arch Internal Medicine* 157 (1997): 2129–36.

Montague, P. "Prescription Drugs That Kill: Another Kind of Drug Problem." *Consumer Law Page,* 2000. <http://consumerlawpage.com/article/drugs_that_kill.shtml>.

Moore, T. "Time to Act on Drug Safety." *JAMA* 279 (May 1998).

Naploi, M. "Some Prescription Drugs Go Over the Counter." *Healthfacts,* August 2000.

National Academy of Sciences. *Report of the International Conference on Adverse Reactions Reporting Systems.* Washington, DC, 1971.

National Center for Health Statistics. "Fast Stats A to Z: Therapeutic Drug Use," August 2001. <http://www.cdc.gov/nchs/fastats/docvisit.htm>.

Neegaard, L. "Irritable Bowel Drug Problem." Associated Press, 31 October 2000. <http://more.abcnews.go.com/sections/living/dailynews/lotronex.html>.

Nelson, K., and R. Talbert, "Drug-Related Hospital Admissions." *Pharmacy Practice Insights,* 1994, 701–7.

Nelson, M., et al. "A Systematic Review of Predictors of Maintenance of Nomotension After Withdrawal of Antihypertensive Drugs." *American Journal of Hypertension* 14 (2001): 98–105.

Oransky, I. "Doctors Step Out; Drug Salesmen Step In." *USA TODAY,* 5 July 2001, 11A.

Orlando, V. "The FDA's Accelerated Approval Process: Does the Pharmaceutical Industry Have Adequate Incentives for Self-Regulation?" *American Journal of Law & Medicine & Ethics* 25 (1999): 543–68.

O'Rourke, K. "AphA McNeil Team Up Against OTC Interactions." *Drug Store News,* 25 October 1999.

Pazart, L. "New Drugs, New Adverse Drug Reactions, and Bibliographic Databases." *Lancet* 353 (1999): 1447–48.

Perz, J., A. Craig, and C. Coffey. "Changes in Antibiotic Prescribing for Children after a Community-Wide Campaign." *JAMA* 287 (2002): 3103–9.

"Phenylpropanolamine Linked to Increased Risk of Stroke." *Medscape News,* 10 November 2000.

Phillips, D., N. Christenfeld, and L. Glynn. "Increase in U.S. Medication-Error Deaths between 1983 and 1993." *Lancet* 351 (1998): 643–44.

Pirmohamed, N, and K. Park. "The Adverse Effects of Drugs." *Hospital Medicine* 60 (1999): 348–52.

"Playing It Safe with Medications." *Janssen Pharmaceutical—Research Foundation,* 2001. <http://www.janssen.com/feature_articles/feature071499.html>.

———. *Prescription Drug User Fee Act, PDUFA Background Information,* 26 July 2000. <http://www.fda.gov/oc/pdufa2/meeting2000/background.html>.

"Prescription Pain-Reliever Duract Recalled Following Four Deaths." *Shawnee News-Star Online,* 23 June 1998. <http://www.news-star.com/stories/062398/lif_prescription.html>.

"Propulsid Used to Treat Babies' Heartburn," *Propulsid Legal Help,* 2000. <www.propulsidlegalhelp.com>.

Pumphrey, R., and S. Davis. "Under-Reporting of Antibiotic Anaphylaxis May Put Patients at Risk." *Lancet* 353 (1999): 1157–58.

Rankin, A. "Non-Sedating Antihistamines and Cardiac Arrhythmia," *Lancet* 350 (1997): 1115–16.

Reh, Maggie, "FDA to Require Pediatric Studies for Drugs Commonly Used in Children." *American Journal Health-Systems Pharmacists* 56 (1999): 203.

———. "Rezulin's Effect on Heart Was Also Seen as Concern." *Los Angeles Times,* 26 March

2000. <http://www.latimes.com/news/nation/reports/rezulin/lat_heart000326.htm>.

———. "The Rise and Fall of the Killer Drug Rezulin." *Los Angeles Times,* 4 June 2000. <http://www.latimes.com/news/nation/reports/rezulin/lat_rezulin000604.htm>.

Rheingold, P. "Ephedra and Other Dangerous Herbals—and Its Cousin PPA." *Rheingold Valet Rheingold & Shkolnik, P.C.,* 343–45.

Rosner, F., et al. "Disclosure and Prevention of Medical Errors." *Arch Internal Medicine* 160 (2000): 2089–92.

Roundtree, R. "Herbs and Drugs for Your Heart: Sorting Out What's Safe." *Herbs for Health* (November/December 1999): 28–29.

Rutherford, E. "The FDA and 'Privatization'—the Drug-Approval Process." *Food and Drug Law Journal,* Anniversary Issue, 203–25.

Schultheis, N. "Propulsid-Related Injuries: What They Are and How to Screen Them."

Schumock, G., and J. Thornton. "Focusing on the Preventability of Adverse Drug Reactions." *American Journal of American Health-System Pharmacists* 27 (1992): 538.

Schwartz, S., et al. "Effect of Troglitazone in Insulin-Treated Patients with Type II Diabetes Mellitus." *New England Journal of Medicine* 338 (March 1998): 861–66.

———. "Second of Two Parts: Drug Maker Hired NIH Researcher." *Los Angeles Times,* 7 December 1998. <http://www.latimes.com/news/nation/reports/rezulin/lat_main981207>.

Smalley, W., et al. "Contraindicated Use of Cisapride." *JAMA* 284 (2000): 3036–39.

Smith, S. "In the News: Dangerous Drug Mishap." *Ladies Home Journal Online,* May 1999. <http://www.findarticles.com/cf_0/ml127/5_116/54515014/pl/article.jhtml>.

Snyderman, N. "Over-the-Counter Danger," *ABCNEWS.com,* 26 May 1999.<http://abcnews.go.com/onair/DailyNews/wnt990526_snyderman_story.html>.

Soumerai, S., et al. "Effect of Government and Commercial Warnings on Reducing Prescription Misuse: The Case of Propoxyphene," *American Journal of Public Health* 77 (1987): 1518–23.

"St. John's Wort." *Drug and Herbal Interactions,* 15 September 2001. <http://www.springnet.com/ce/cam_mod2s07.htm>.

Sternberg, S. "Lawsuits: Drug Development's Side Effect." *USA Today,* 12 January 2000.

Thomas, E. "Incidence and Types of Preventable Adverse Events in Elderly Patients: Population Based Review of Medical Records." *British Medical Journal* 320 (2000): 741–44.

Thompson, L. "User Fees for Faster Drug Reviews: Are They Helping or Hurting the Public Health?" *FDA Consumer Magazine,* September–October 2000. <http://www.fda.gov/fdacfeatures/2000/500_pdufa.html>.

Tobias, D., and C. Pulliam. "General and Psychotherapeutic Medication Use in 878 Nursing Facilities: A 1997 National Survey." *Consultant Pharmacist* 12 (1997): 1401–8.

U.S. Food and Drug Administration Center for Drug Evaluation and Research. *New Drug Development and Review Process,* 2000. <http://www.fda.gov/cder/handbook/dev_rev.htm>.

U.S. Food and Drug Administration. *Consumer Special Report: Benefit vs. Risk: How CDER Approves Drugs,* January 1995.

———. "Warning About Mixing Prescription Drugs Not Always Given." *Atlanta Journal Constitution*, 19 August 1996. <http://www.pendulum.org/articles/mising_meds.htm>.

Watkins, P. B., and R. W. Whitcomb. "Hepatic Dysfunction Associated with Troglitazone." *New England Journal of Medicine,* 916–17, Letter to the Editor, 26 March 1998.

BIBLIOGRAPHY

Weber, T. "Emerging Antibiotic Resistance." *American College of Physicians— American Society of Internal Medicine,* Diss. 2000 Annual Session Press Briefing, 14 April 2000. <http://www.acponline.org/ear/weber.htm>.

White, T., A. Arakelian, and J. Rho. "Counting the Costs of Drug-Related Adverse Events." *Pharmacoeconomics* 15 (1999): 445–58.

Willis, J. "Using Over-the-Counter Medication Wisely." *FDA Consumer Magazine,* November 1991. <http://www.uark.edu/depts/healinfo/otcs.htm>.

Willman, David, "Drug After Drug, Warnings Ignored." *Los Angeles Times Health: Consumer,* 20 December 2000. <http://www.latimes.com/health/consumer/connews/20001220/t000121358.html>.

Woodcock, J. "An FDA Perspective on the Drug Development Process." *Food and Drug Law Journal* 52 (1997): 145–50.

Zevitas, Christa. "Diabetes Drug Could Spur Next Big Pharmaceutical Litigation." *Lawyers Weekly, Inc.,* 12 April 2001. <http://www.lweekly.com/diabetes.cfm>.

Index

Accupril, 99
ACE inhibitors
  complications with, 205
  and high blood pressure, 10–11,
    99–100, 132
  and physician communication, 199
acetaminophen, 85, 159–162, 171
Achilles tendon, 206
acid reflux, 76–78, 81, 211
AIDS, 31–35, 59. *See also* HIV
Aleve, 86, 114, 161
Alexander, Dr. Duane, 40–41
allergies, 138, 180
allergist, 131
Alliance for the Prudent Use of
  Antibiotics, 126
Altace, 99
alpha-lipoic acid, 229
Alzheimer's dementia
  cause of, 178
  and hormone replacement therapy, 4
  medication for, 58, 138
  and nutritional supplements, 226–27
American Academy of Family
  Practice, 126
American Academy of Pediatrics, 40, 126
American Academy Society for
  Microbiology, 126
American Journal of Hypertension, 211
amoxicillin, 204
ampicillin, 204
anaphylactic reaction, 203
angioplasty, 134
angiotensin converting enzyme inhibitors.
  See ACE inhibitors
angiotensin II antagonists, 99–100
antibiotics
  for acute treatment, 201
  bacterial resistance to, 124–127
  for bronchitis, 206
  and drug interactions, 149, 159

fluroquinolone, 141–42
antidepressant, 187–88, 190
antifungal, 149
antihistamine, 116, 149, 169
antioxidant, 227–29
anxiety, 133, 138–39
appendicitis, 216
Archives of Internal Medicine, 127
arrhythmia, 50
arthritis
  cause of, 178
  and drug effectiveness, 26, 132–33
  essential fats and, 221
  medication, 138, 171–72
  and nutritional supplements, 145, 189,
    226–27
aspirin, 114, 137, 145, 171, 188
asthma, 26, 138, 221, 228
Atacand, 100
atenolol, 205
Ativan, 189–90
atrial fibrillation, 134–35, 153
autoimmune diseases, 221
Avapro, 100
Axid, 137, 161
AZT, 33

bacterial resistance, 125
Bates, Dr. David, 12, 123
Baycol, 91–100, 199
Bedell, Dr. Susanna, 127
Benicar, 100
beta-blocker, 132
Betapace, 128–29, 135, 144
birth defects, 21–22
black cohosh, 188
black box warning, 50, 82–84, 95
Blackburn, Dr. George, 167
Blackburn-Morgan study, 167
bladder infection, 176

252

About the Author

RAY D. STRAND, M.D., GRADUATED FROM THE UNIVERSITY OF
Colorado Medical School and finished his postgraduate training at
Mercy Hospital in San Diego, California. He has been involved in an
active private family practice for the past thirty years. He has focused
his practice on nutritional medicine over the past seven years while lec-
turing internationally on the subject and is the author of *What Your
Doctor Doesn't Know About Nutritional Medicine May Be Killing You*. Dr.
Strand lives on a horse ranch in South Dakota with his lovely wife,
Elizabeth. They have three grown children.

For more information on Dr. Strand's consulting and speaking services, you can contact Dr. Strand at:

> Ray D. Strand, M.D.
> P. O. Box 9226
> Rapid City, SD 57709

> Visit Dr. Strand's website:
> www.drraystrand.com

Acknowledgments

AFTER THIS, MY SECOND BOOK, I KNOW WITHOUT A DOUBT that only a team of players makes the writing process possible. I'd like to thank those whose names I know, and those behind the scenes who believed in and participated in the writing of this book.

First, to my agent, Chip MacGregor, and the entire staff at Alive Communications, who have guided me impeccably, thank you. A thousand thanks belong to Alice Crider, who always takes time to listen, making sure everything is well tended. Also a huge thanks for the index, figures, and tables.

I have been most fortunate to be published by Thomas Nelson. Victor Oliver and Michael Hyatt's ideas, wisdom, and support have been tremendous. This manuscript has been in the best of hands with Kristen Lucas, my managing editor; Pamela Clements, the vice president of marketing; and the entire staff at Thomas Nelson.

Throughout this project I have felt like an investigative reporter. You might think a physician would know everything needed about the drug-approval process and adverse side effects of the drugs he prescribes. Nothing could be further from the truth. Thank you, Verne Goodsell, Tom Simmons, Leone Young, and Karmen Thompson for helping me gather all the research necessary for a book of this caliber.

I want to give special thanks to my collaborator, Donna Wallace, whose talent and energy made this project a reality. I realize the facts and concepts presented in this book will help thousands of people; however, it is the writing talent of Donna Wallace that will keep you turning its pages. I also want to express my personal thanks to Donna's mother, Barbara Ward, for the fine polish she brought to the text by hours of meticulous care in proofreading.

Finally, my deepest gratitude goes to Elizabeth, my love and inspiration. Behind every moment of my success stand the faith and undying support of my wife. Liz, your passion and determination to live well restores my belief in God while renewing my faith in the apex of His creation, the human body. I am truly blessed.

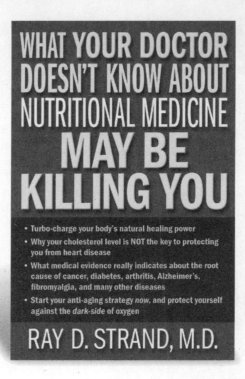

WHAT YOUR DOCTOR DOESN'T KNOW ABOUT NUTRITIONAL MEDICINE MAY BE KILLING YOU

- Turbo-charge your body's natural healing power
- Why your cholesterol level is NOT the key to protecting you from heart disease
- What medical evidence really indicates about the root cause of cancer, diabetes, arthritis, Alzheimer's, fibromyalgia, and many other diseases
- Start your anti-aging strategy *now*, and protect yourself against the *dark-side* of oxygen

RAY D. STRAND, M.D.

When Dr. Ray Strand found himself in a losing battle, unable to successfully treat his wife, who had suffered chronically with pain and fatigue, he agreed to have her try the regimen of nutritional supplements that a neighbor suggested. Much to his surprise, his wife's condition began to improve almost immediately, and now she enjoys a full life with excellent health. That amazing turn of events led him to dedicate himself to researching alternative therapies in medicine, particularly in the arena of nutritional supplements.

Dr. Strand's illumination of the body's silent enemy—oxidative stress—will astound you. But, more importantly, his research will equip you to protect or reclaim your nutritional health, possibly reversing disease and preventing illness.

ISBN: 0-7852-6486-8